Shared Care for
Osteoporosis

Shared Care for Osteoporosis

Roger Smith MA MD PhD FRCP
Consultant Physician, Nuffield Orthopaedic Centre,
Headington, Oxford, UK

John Harrison MBBS MRCP MRCGP DRCOG DFFP
General Practitioner, Washington House Surgery,
Brackley, Northamptonshire, UK

Cyrus Cooper MA DM FRCP
MRC Clinical Scientist, Professor of Rheumatology and
Consultant Rheumatologist,
MRC Environmental Epidemiology Unit,
University of Southampton,
Southampton General Hospital,
Southampton, UK

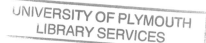
**I S I S
MEDICAL
M E D I A**

Oxford

© 1998 Isis Medical Media Ltd
59 St Aldates
Oxford OX1 1ST, UK

First published 1998

British Library Cataloguing in Publication Data
A catalogue record for this title is available from the British Library

ISBN 1 899066 26 8

Smith, R. (Roger)
Shared Care for Osteoporosis
Roger Smith, John Harrison and Cyrus Cooper

Always refer to the manufacturer's Prescribing Information before prescribing drugs cited in this book.

Typeset by
Creative Associates, Oxford, UK

Produced by Phoenix Offset,HK
Printed in Hong Kong

Distributed in the USA by
Mosby-Year Book Inc., 11830 Westline Industrial Drive,
St. Louis, Mo 63145, USA

Distributed in the rest of the world by
Plymbridge Distributors Ltd, Estover Road,
Plymouth PL6 7PY, UK

Contents

Acknowledgements

We are indebted to our families for their patience, to our secretaries for their tolerance and to Julian Grover for his considerable efforts.

Preface

The main aim of this book is to improve the management of patients with, or likely to develop, osteoporosis. It is intended as a practical guide for all health professionals involved in shared patient care.

The introductory sections explain the ways in which osteoporosis develops and describe the nature and extent of the problem. Subsequent chapters discuss diagnosis, methods of prevention and treatment. Current problems are then dealt with as well as the optimal structure for shared care.

Although we have attempted to keep repetition to a minimum, some topics, particularly densitometry and hormone replacement therapy, are of primary importance and are covered in several chapters in the text. Several comprehensive reviews have been published recently and the authors have referred the interested reader to these, where appropriate, thus avoiding long reference lists at the end of each chapter.

Each contributing author is a specialist concerned with a different aspect of osteoporosis and we hope that our personal experience and insight into the field has been an advantage when writing about a disease which involves a wide range of clinical specialities.

R. Smith, J. Harrison, C. Cooper

Chapter 1

Introduction

Introduction

Osteoporosis is a condition that has recently assumed great importance. A number of factors have contributed to this; they are summarized in this chapter and subsequently in more detail in Chapter 3. Osteoporosis is not a new disease but it is largely related to age, and increased life expectancy is the main reason why it is now more common than in previous centuries.

Current interest in osteoporosis arises from the recognition that it contributes significantly to bony fragility and fracture, that the likelihood of fracture may now be predicted, and that the prevention and treatment of osteoporosis should significantly reduce fracture rate.

Such a reduction would have enormous potential benefits both to affected persons and to the health service. The development of drugs effective in the prevention of bone loss also holds the promise of large financial rewards for the pharmaceutical industry and drives much current research. The problems of osteoporosis are by no means solved (Chapter 7) and new knowledge continues to appear.

Shared care

For the full advantages of current work on osteoporosis to be made available to patients, it is important that this knowledge should be widely disseminated to those who have the responsibility for their care. The main aim of this book is to provide such a review of current knowledge. A particularly valuable UK document is the 1994 Department of Health Advisory Group's *Report on Osteoporosis*, the AGO report[1]. Other very recent sources include the books by Rosen[2], by Kanis[3] and by Marcus, Feldman and Kelsey[4]; the first two provide useful clinical advice and the third also deals comprehensively with normal and abnormal bone physiology.

History

Current research suggests that osteoporosis is not a new disease, and that bone loss has always occurred with age, although its rate may have accelerated[5]. Astley Cooper[6], Albright and Reifenstein[7] and Cooke[8] gave early and full descriptions of the loss of bone and consequent fractures, especially of the hip, in elderly women.

For those interested in the skeleton, the causes of osteoporosis have long been controversial. In particular, the question as to whether calcium loss in postmenopausal women is a cause or result of osteoporosis has been pursued with much energy but little success.

The changing view of osteoporosis, from a disease that is suitable only for academic argument to one that is of outstanding importance in the real world, has come particularly from the increase in fractures as the population ages.

Whether age-related bone loss is physiological or pathological is largely irrelevant. What is of critical importance is that the reduction in the amount of bone, loosely referred to as 'bone density', and the increasing fragility that ensues, contribute to the exponential increase in disabling and potentially life-threatening fractures[1].

Osteoporosis and fracture

The relationship of osteoporosis to fracture, together with the likely causes of their increased incidence, are dealt with in Chapter 3. An outstanding question in this area is how much the loss of bone (and its architectural deterioration) contributes to the increase in fracture rate. Since fracture rate increases as bone mass falls and, less convincingly, declines when bone loss is prevented, there is clearly a close relationship between the two. Although measured bone mass is the most useful available predictor of individual fracture risk, there is, in populations, an overlap in bone density between those who fracture and those who do not. This implies that there are other important determinants of fracture, of which the increasing tendency to fall with advancing age is probably the most significant (Chapter 3).

Bone density

Nevertheless, modern densitometric methods utilizing dual X-ray absorptiometry (DXA) (Chapter 4) have made it possible to predict fracture risk and to provide a quantitative measurement of the effects of treatment (Chapters 5 and 6). Densitometry is also valuable in research (Chapter 7). Assessment of the skeletal effects of bone-active drugs and other preventative measures is most often made by measurement of bone density. In particular, the prevention of bone loss is regularly used as a surrogate for a reduction in fracture rate, although this is not universally acceptable. The problems surrounding this assumption are discussed in subsequent chapters.

Financial burdens

The population costs of osteoporosis-related fractures are very difficult to assess, although the personal cost is undoubted. Apart from the fact that it is impossible to know how much osteoporosis contributes to fracture, it is also difficult to assess the long-term (rather than the early) financial cost. Estimates (Chapter 3) often assume that all hip fractures over the age of 65 are due to osteoporosis, which is unlikely, but do include the large cost of institutional care, which is a very important component of the financial burden.

The total estimated annual 'osteoporosis' cost to the UK of more than £900 million clearly constitutes a large health service bill; if it were possible to reduce this significantly, by decreasing bone loss and reducing fracture rate, this would lead to considerable financial savings. How far a reduction of bone loss (or the 10% increase in bone density that is all that is likely to be achieved by current treatment) will in itself produce a worthwhile reduction in fracture rate remains largely unknown.

The patient

With regard to the individual patient, with whom this book is largely concerned, any measures that reduce bone loss and hence the likelihood of osteoporosis-related fractures — especially of the hip — are clearly worthwhile. These can be in the area of basic bone biology, in therapeutic development and in shared care (Chapter 8). Since falls are an important contributor to fracture, the causes and prevention of these must also be fully considered.

Key points

■ With increasing longevity, age-related bone loss contributing to fracture has become a major medical problem.

■ It is now possible to measure bone mass accurately, to predict the likelihood of fracture, to prevent and treat osteoporosis and to reduce fracture frequency.

■ The potential benefits of this to the health service, to the pharmaceutical industry (which develops the osteotropic agents) and, most importantly, to the patient, are considerable.

■ These benefits are best brought to the individual by a system of shared health care.

References

1 Advisory Group on Osteoporosis. *Report on Osteoporosis*. Wetherby: Department of Health, 1994.

2 Rosen CJ. *Osteoporosis. Diagnostic and Therapeutic Principles*. Totowa: Humana Press, 1996.

3 Kanis JA. *Osteoporosis*. Oxford: Blackwell, 1994.

4 Marcus R, Feldman D, Kelsey J, eds. *Osteoporosis*. New York: Academic Press, 1996.

5 Lees B, Molleson T, Arnett TR, Stevenson JC. Differences in proximal femur bone density over two centuries. *Lancet* 1993; **341**: 673–5.

6 Cooper A. *A Treatise on Dislocations and Fractures of the Joints*, 6th Edn. London: Longman Rees; Orme Brown; Highley; Underwood, 1829.

7 Albright F, Reifenstein EC. *The Parathyroid Glands and Metabolic Bone Disease.* Baltimore: Williams and Wilkins, 1948.

8 Cooke AM. Osteoporosis. *Lancet* 1955; i: 877–92, 929–37.

Chapter 2

Life cycle of the skeleton

Introduction

Bone is a metabolically active tissue that is formed, removed and replaced throughout life. Mineralization of its organic matrix produces a tissue of considerable strength and provides the body's store of calcium; this also accounts for the persistence of bone after death and the erroneous impression that it is inert. To understand osteoporosis it is essential to review the structure and physiology of bone, which centre around the activity of its specialized cells[1-8].

Bone as a tissue

The main structural components of bone are the organic matrix, composed predominantly of collagen (a heteropolymeric triple helical molecule arranged in strong fibres), and a mineral (hydroxyapatite), which is laid down upon this matrix in an organized manner by the bone-forming cells, the osteoblasts (Figure 2.1). In the adult skeleton two main anatomical forms of bone are recognized — cortical and trabecular (spongy). The cortical form is composed of tightly packed mineralized bone organized into Haversian systems; these are cylindrical units of compact bone structure built around a central, vascular canal and composed of concentric bony lamellae. Cortical bone is largely constructed on the outside shell of the long bones to provide strength on the perimeter of the cylinder. Trabecular bone has a porous sponge-like structure in which trabeculae of bone are joined to each other in the form of a three-dimensional mesh

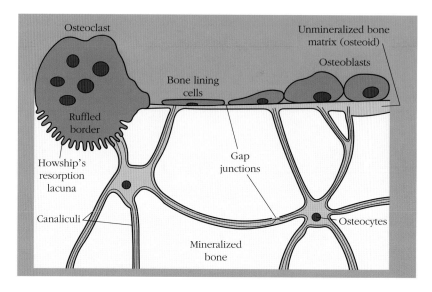

Figure 2.1 *A diagram to show the main components of bone. (Based on ref. 1, Oxford University Press, with permission.)*

enclosing elements of the bone marrow. This form of bone is found in the vertebral bodies, in particular. The turnover rate of trabecular bone is more rapid than that of cortical bone, owing to its relatively greater surface area; this is one reason why the loss of bone (for instance, after the menopause) is earliest and most rapid in the spine.

Components of bone

The main components of bone are the organic matrix, bone mineral and bone cells. Organic components of the bone matrix may be divided into collagen and non-collagen protein, as follows:

- Type I collagen (95%)
- Non-collagen substances (5%)
  - proteoglycan
  - osteonectin
  - sialoprotein
  - osteocalcin
  - bone morphogenetic proteins.

There is a large family of genetically different collagens with different structures appropriate to their functions[9]. The most abundant fibrillar collagen and the main collagen of bone is type I.

Collagen is synthesized by the osteoblasts, which are also responsible for its mineralization and which interact with the bone-resorbing cells, the osteoclasts. The osteoblasts are derived from cells of the stromal system, the pre-osteoblasts, and are the precursors of the osteocytes which are found in the mineralized bone. Current evidence suggests that the osteocytes are important as the main route by which mechanical signals induce new bone formation.

Bone matrix

Collagen

Collagen, the major extracellular protein in the body, comprises a large family with the common feature of a repetitive Gly-X-Y (gly = glycine, X and Y are often proline and hydroxyproline, respectively) sequence. This molecular structure allows the constituent α-chains to arrange themselves in the form of a triple helix with glycine at its centre, and to form intramolecular and intermolecular crosslinks. The resultant fibres have astonishing tensile strength, provided that the molecular structure (and the subsequent crosslinking) is accurate (Figure 2.2).

Most type I collagen is in the skeleton but it is also found in other tissues, largely on its own (as in tendons and sclerae) and sometimes with other collagens — such as type III in the skin. The relevance of collagen to osteoporosis is as follows:

- it contributes to the strength of bone
- mutations in the genes for type I collagen cause bone fragility (osteogenesis imperfecta)
- it is possible that collagen may sometimes be abnormal in osteoporosis
- collagen forms a basis for mineralization, and
- measurement of its circulating or excreted breakdown products give an indication of bone turnover and resorption.

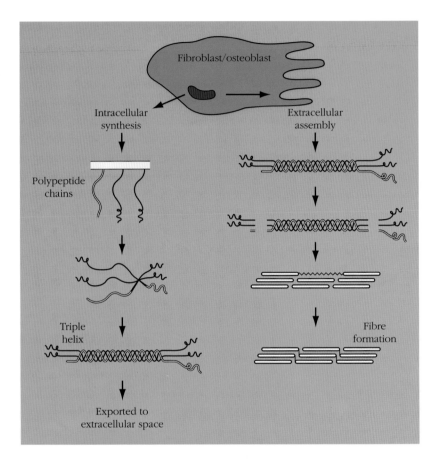

Figure 2.2 *The synthesis and structure of type I collagen. The polypeptide (α) chains are synthesized and modified within the cell to form a triple helical molecule that is exported and aggregates into the collagen fibre. (Based on ref. I, Oxford University Press, with permission.)*

Non-collagen proteins

The skeleton contains numerous non-collagen protein constituents, the function of which is largely unknown; these include the sialoproteins, phosphoproteins and numerous others[6], including proteoglycans[10]. For many years it has been known that extracts of demineralized bone can induce ectopic ossification, particularly in muscle. The substances that bring this about have now been identified as a family of bone morphogenetic proteins (BMPs)[11]. These proteins:

■ are a unique subfamily of transforming growth factor (TGF)β proteins
■ induce ectopic bone
■ influence the pattern of early skeletal development.

The genes for BMPs are related to the large gene family that codes for the TGFβ proteins and also for the proteins concerned with limb patterning and development. These discoveries are of considerable biological importance as they suggest ways in which the amount of bone within the normal skeleton may be influenced.

Bone mineral

There appear to be two different ways in which bone becomes mineralized. In the first, mineral is laid down in association with very small mineralizing vesicles apparently derived from osteoblasts (or chondroblasts). These vesicles contain, and presumably produce, alkaline phosphatase. This enzyme is also a pyrophosphatase and it has been proposed that the breakdown of pyrophosphate (which normally inhibits mineralization) allows mineralization to occur. This system, centred around calcifying vesicles, occurs particularly in the preliminary ossification of cartilage and foetal bone. In mature bone a second mechanism probably predominates. This relies on a template of collagen fibres, which are arranged in a three-dimensional quarter-stagger array that provides regularly alternating gaps or hole zones (Figure 2.3). Observation of experimental systems such as calcifying turkey tendons shows the precision of this process. However, despite many suggestions, the exact biochemical basis for mineralization is unknown. It is clear that bone mineral, which is a complex crystalline structure known as hydroxyapatite, adds strength and rigidity to the collagen matrix. In conditions such as rickets and osteomalacia, where mineralization is defective, bone loses its rigidity and is easily deformed. Likewise, where the collagen matrix is faulty, as in osteogenesis imperfecta, the skeleton is excessively fragile.

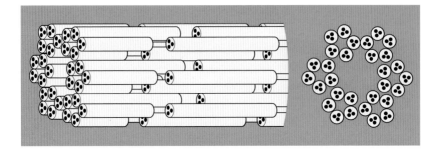

Figure 2.3 *Three-dimensional quarter-stagger array of collagen molecules. Mineralization begins in the gap zones, later extending to the overlap zones.*

Bone cells

Bone contains specific cells, the osteoblasts, osteoclasts and osteocytes, which are in close association with the bone marrow and the cells of the haemopoietic system (Figure 2.4).

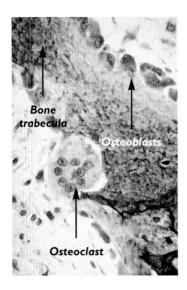

Figure 2.4 *Histological section of bone to show osteoblasts and a multinucleated osteoclast (arrowed).*

The osteoblast

The osteoblast is essential for bone formation and lies at the centre of bone physiology (Figure 2.5). It synthesizes bone collagen, non-collagen proteins and alkaline phosphatase and controls mineralization. It also controls the activity of the osteoclasts by mechanisms that are not understood.

The function and behaviour of the osteoblasts depend on many factors. These include genetic, mechanical, nutritional and endocrine influences, as well as the effect of local chemical messages produced by the cells — the cytokines (see the section on 'bone cell conversation', pages 16–17).

■ Bone mass (and presumably osteoblast function; see also below) is heritable and differs with family, race, collagen gene mutations and possibly changes in the vitamin D receptor.

■ Mechanical stress stimulates osteoblast function in experimental systems and bone is formed along the lines of stress (Wolff's law), but the mechanisms are unknown. It is possible that osteocytes provide the link that transforms mechanical into biological systems in bone.

■ The effects of nutritional and endocrine factors on the osteoblast are complex. Although bone size and mass are greater in those who are properly nourished and have a high calcium intake, the reasons for this are not known.

■ Amongst endocrine factors, the sex hormones and calciotropic hormones are particularly important. Testosterone lack in men and oestrogen lack in women reduce bone mass but, again, the mechanisms are not well understood. Osteoblasts contain oestrogen receptors but only a few.

■ In experimental systems, parathyroid hormone (and some derivatives of it) initially stimulate osteoblast activity. Corticosteroids suppress the activity of the osteoblasts and growth hormone stimulates it.

■ Finally, the osteoblast appears to act as an intermediate between various hormone systems and the osteoclast.

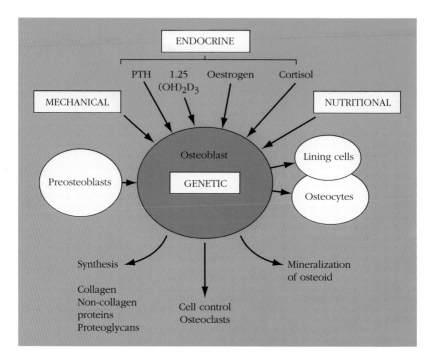

Figure 2.5 *The central position of the osteoblast in bone physiology. Important factors which control bone mass are in capitals. (Based on ref. 1, Oxford University Press, with permission.)*

The osteoclast

The osteoclast is a multinucleated cell derived from precursors within the haemopoietic system. It is a specialized bone-resorbing cell that seals off an area of the bone surface to produce a very acid environment within which its lysosomal enzymes resorb whole bone. The hydrogen ions necessary for this activity are produced by the carbonic anhydrase system (Figure 2.6). Absence of this enzyme causes a rare form of osteopetrosis (marble bone disease) because bone resorption is defective; other defects of osteoclast function may lead to osteopetrosis in humans and animals. Calcitonin directly suppresses the osteoclast. Current evidence suggests that the effects of other hormones, such as parathyroid hormone, which increase bone resorption, are mediated via the osteoblast.

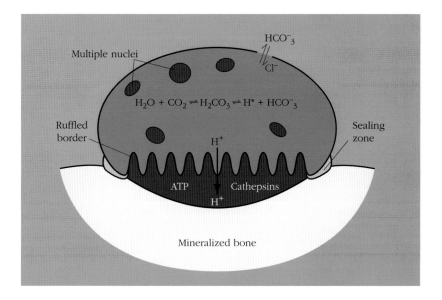

Figure 2.6 *Important features of the osteoclast. Resorption occurs within the acid sealed zone. (Based on ref. 1, Oxford University Press, with permission.)*

The osteocyte

The osteocyte, derived from the osteoblast, lies within mineralized bone and communicates with its neighbours through its extensions in the canaliculi. This cell may detect mechanical deformation and mediate the osteoblast response to this.

Bone multicellular units

The skeleton is constantly being resorbed and rebuilt by teams of bone cells. In youth these processes favour synthesis; in old age they favour resorption. The cellular system around which this balance is centred is the bone multicellular unit (BMU; also known as the bone remodelling unit, BRU). There are innumerable BMUs on the surface of trabecular bone and within the cortex, which are at different stages in their life cycle. This cycle begins with the activation of bone resorption and ends with the replacement of bone by osteoblasts

(Figure 2.7). These cycles may each take up to 6 months (Figure 2.8). The possible therapeutic manipulation of BMUs is important in considering how bone loss may be prevented or bone mass increased. This is likely to be more effective in the young skeleton than in the old, because of the larger number of active BMUs in youth.

Bone cell conversation

There is good evidence to suggest that the activities of the osteoblasts and osteoclasts are normally closely linked under physiological and pathological conditions (for instance in Paget's disease) but the mechanisms for the linkage are not understood. Bone cells (and other cells) produce a great variety of locally acting cell-derived substances called cytokines, which can be shown to have many different actions in experimental systems.

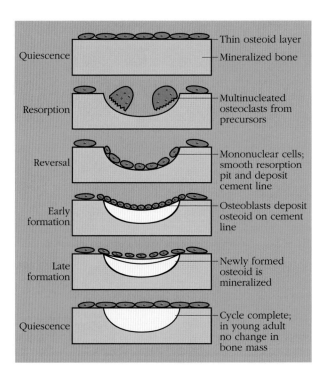

Figure 2.7
Changes that occur in the bone multicellular unit (BMU). This represents the surface of trabecular bone; similar changes occur in the cortical bone. (Based on ref. 1, Oxford University Press, with permission.)

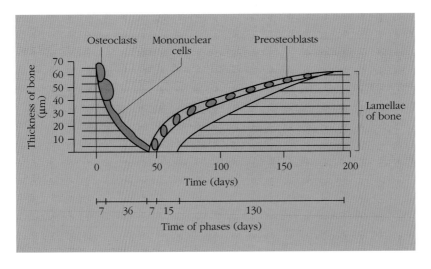

Figure 2.8 *Estimated time-scale of a bone-remodelling cycle. (Based on ref. 1, Oxford University Press, with permission.)*

The major cytokines comprise:

- interleukins
- tumour necrosis factors
- interferons
- growth factors
- colony-stimulating factors.

The physiological function of the cytokines is largely unknown[7,12].

One particular problem is how the BMU cycle begins. There is some evidence that the osteoblast produces osteoclast-activating factors (OAFs); there is also some evidence that the resorption of bone may release biologically active bone mitogenic substances that turn on osteoblastic activity.

Calcium and phosphate balance

The central position of calcium as an ionic messenger continues to be explored. It is essential for innumerable functions such as reproduction, neurotransmission, hormone action, cellular growth and enzyme action. There have been considerable advances in our understanding of the messengers that control cellular processes by generating internal calcium signals. Chief amongst these is inositol triphosphate, which is generated via G-protein and tyrosine kinase-linked receptors.

Much is now known about external calcium balance and the main hormones that control it; phosphate balance is less well understood. The circulating concentration of plasma calcium is determined by the amount of calcium absorbed by the intestine, the amount excreted by the kidney, and the exchange of mineral with the skeleton. The relative importance of these exchanges differs during growth and pregnancy and in different disorders. Total plasma calcium is closely maintained between 2.25 and 2.60 mmol/l, of which nearly half is in the ionized form (47% ionized, 46% protein bound, and the remainder complexed). The skeleton contains approximately 1 kg (25,000 mmol) of calcium. The main daily fluxes of calcium in the adult are shown in Figure 2.9.

Parathyroid hormone (PTH)

The gene for PTH is on chromosome 11. The hormone is synthesized as a large precursor like other proteins packaged for export. Its secretion is stimulated by a reduction in the plasma concentration of ionized calcium. Parathyroid cells respond to changes in the extracellular concentration of calcium via a recently identified calcium-sensing receptor.

An increase in PTH leads to an increase in calcium absorption through the gut, in calcium reabsorption through the kidney, and in bone resorption. Intestinal calcium absorption is mediated by the active metabolite of vitamin D, 1,25-dihydroxycholecalciferol (1,25-$(OH)_2D_3$). In contrast, the effect of parathyroid hormone on renal calcium reabsorption is direct. The cellular effects of PTH on kidney and bone appear to utilize more than one system. PTH encourages osteoclastic bone resorption by its effects on the osteoblast, as previously described.

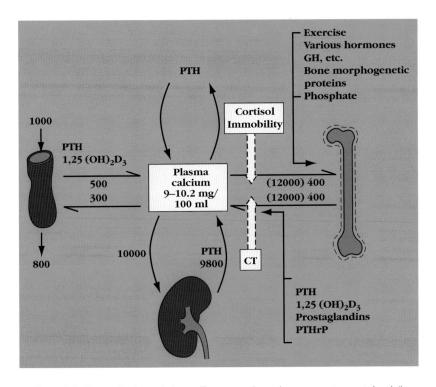

Figure 2.9 *External calcium balance. The numerals on the arrows represent the daily movements (mg/day) in the adult (those in parentheses indicate the possible exchange through the bone cell envelope (dotted arrows)). PTH = parathyroid hormone; PTHrP = parathyroid hormone-related peptide; CT = calcitonin; GH = growth hormone. (Based on ref. 1, Oxford University Press, with permission.)*

Vitamin D

Vitamin D is synthesized either as vitamin D_3 (cholecalciferol) within the skin from its precursor 7-dehydrocholesterol under the influence of ultraviolet light (usually as sunlight), or taken in with food, either as vitamin D_3 or D_2 (ergocalciferol) (Figure 2.10). It is subsequently transported to the liver by a binding protein where it undergoes 25-hydroxylation; 25-hydroxyvitamin D (25(OH)D) is then hydroxylated in the 1 position by the renal 1α-hydroxylase. The classic action of the active metabolite, $1,25(OH)_2D$, is on calcium metabolism, promoting

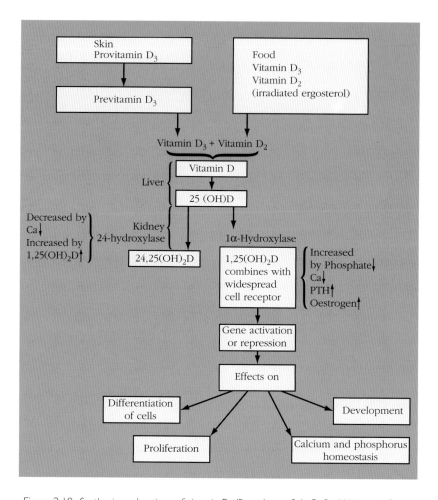

Figure 2.10 *Synthesis and actions of vitamin D. (Based on ref. 1, Oxford University Press, with permission.)*

the synthesis of a calcium-transporting protein within the cells of the small intestine. Its effects are mediated through a widely distributed vitamin D receptor with DNA and hormone-binding components[13].

It is now known that $1,25(OH)_2D$ has many effects outside mineral metabolism, concerned with the immune system and the growth and differentiation of a wide variety of cells.

Measurement of plasma 25(OH)D has proved to be a useful indicator of vitamin D status and work on 1,25(OH)$_2$D and its receptors has identified the causes of the rarer forms of inherited rickets.

Although the kidney is the main source of 1,25(OH)$_2$D, this metabolite can also be synthesized by a variety of granulomata, which provides a partial explanation for the hypercalcaemia of sarcoidosis and (occasionally) lymphomas.

Some, but not all, work suggests that bone mass is partly linked to certain polymorphic changes in the vitamin D receptor gene[14].

Calcitonin

The main effect of administered calcitonin is to reduce bone resorption by direct and reversible suppression of the osteoclast. The physiological role of calcitonin is uncertain, although it is thought to protect the skeleton during such stresses as growth and pregnancy.

Parathyroid hormone-related protein (PTHrP)

The hormone PTHrP was discovered during studies on patients with non-metastatic hypercalcaemia of malignancy. It has close sequence homology with PTH at the amino-terminal end of the molecule and has very similar effects. Its gene is on the short arm of chromosome 12, thought to have arisen by a duplication of chromosome 11, which carries the human PTH gene. It has been detected in a number of tumours, particularly of the lung. There is also evidence that it may have a role in foetal physiology, controlling the calcium gradient across the placenta and maintaining the relatively higher concentrations in the foetal circulation, and in cartilage development.

Other hormones

Apart from the recognized calciotropic hormones, the skeleton is influenced by corticosteroids, the sex hormones, thyroxine, and growth hormone, as follows:

- excess corticosteroids (either therapeutic or in Cushing's disease) suppress osteoblastic new bone formation,
- both androgens and oestrogens promote and maintain skeletal mass; osteoblasts have receptors for oestrogens, although they are not abundant,
- thyroxine increases bone turnover and increases resorption in excess of formation; thyrotoxicosis thus reduces bone mass, and
- excess growth hormone leads to gigantism and acromegaly (according to the age of onset) with enlargement of the bones; absence of growth hormone will lead to proportional short stature; where there is wider pituitary failure, the reduction in gonadotrophins will cause bone loss.

Biochemical measurements of bone cell activity

Knowledge of bone physiology enables biochemical measures of bone turnover to be interpreted (Figure 2.11). Such measures include the plasma bone-derived alkaline phosphatase and osteocalcin, and urinary total hydroxyproline and crosslinked collagen-derived peptides. The first two of these are closely related to osteoblast function, and the second two to bone resorption. As formation and resorption are closely coupled, such measurements are usually also closely related to each other, and to overall bone turnover.

Plasma alkaline phosphatase (largely derived from osteoblasts) provides a reliable and readily accessible index of bone formation, being increased during periods of rapid growth and particularly where bone turnover is greatly increased, as in Paget's disease; where more skeletal specificity is required, measurement of bone-derived (rather than total) alkaline phosphatase can be useful.

- Early measurements of serum osteocalcin (bone Gla protein) were widely variable and depended on the origin, sensitivity and stability of the antibodies used.

- Total urine hydroxyproline is influenced by dietary collagen (gelatin) and reflects both resorption and new collagen synthesis.

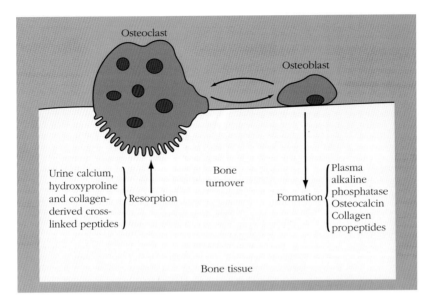

Figure 2.11 *Origin of biochemical indicators of bone cell activity.*

■ The recent development of methods for the measurement of urinary collagen-derived pyridinium crosslinks promises to give a reliable indication of bone resorption unrelated to new collagen formation and uninfluenced by diet[15]. This may be particularly useful in detecting the suppression of bone resorption by the newly available anti-resorptive bisphosphonates such as alendronate (see Chapter 6).

■ Other research methods include measurement of circulating fragments of the collagen molecule derived from its carboxy-terminal and amino-terminal extensions which, under certain circumstances, indicate the rate of collagen (bone) formation.

Metabolic bone diseases

The correct diagnosis of osteoporosis requires an understanding of other metabolic bone diseases. These are largely explained by the normal physiology of bone. They may be inherited or acquired and common or rare, and are usefully classified into the classic metabolic bone diseases (osteoporosis, osteomalacia, Paget's disease, parathyroid bone disease and neoplastic bone disease) and the more recently identified disorders of bone matrix (such as osteogenesis imperfecta, achondroplasia and Marfan's syndrome), the biochemical basis of which is now known. These are dealt with in larger texts and summarized in Table 2.1.

Table 2.1 Main features and causes of some metabolic bone diseases

Disease	Main features	Main biochemical changes	Main cause
Osteoporosis	Fracture	Normal	Oestrogen lack
Osteomalacia	Deformity Myopathy	Low plasma calcium	Vitamin D deficiency or resistance
Parathyroid bone disease	Bone pain Fracture	High plasma calcium	Parathyroid adenoma
Paget's disease	Deformity Fracture	High plasma alkaline phosphatase	Possible virus
Osteogenesis imperfecta	Fractures	Normal	Type I collagen gene mutations
Marfan's syndrome	Disproportion Dissecting aorta Dislocated lenses	Normal	Fibrillin gene mutations
Achondroplasia	Short stature	Normal	Fibroblast growth factor receptor 3 gene mutations

Bone mass

Major determinants

The main determinants of bone mass are those that influence the balance between osteoblast and osteoclast activity — namely, the interaction between genetic and mechanical factors, modified by nutritional and endocrine influences. These have been considered previously and some examples are shown in Figure 2.12. Recent research has failed to establish any single clear cause of the difference between the bone mass of adult Whites and Blacks and of Caucasians and Orientals. The combined effect of malnutrition and oestrogen deficiency in anorexia nervosa has received much attention. Likewise, obsessional exercise associated with oestrogen lack is a recognised cause of low bone mass in females, whereas in those who are not hormone deficient the beneficial effect of mechanical stress on the skeleton continues to be confirmed.

Change with age

There are well-defined changes in the skeleton with age (Figure 2.13). During the growth of childhood and adolescence, bone mass (in grams of calcium) and size increase. Bone mineral density (BMD) expressed as gCa/cm^2, also increases (Chapter 4). BMD in this form is not corrected for the continuing true increase in size, since it is expressed in terms of an area, and it is therefore difficult to interpret changes in BMD with age[16]. However, quantitative computerized tomography (QCT) measurements of bone density are volumetric.

From the age of 25–35 years the BMD is at its maximum; this value is referred to as the peak bone mass.

From 35–40 years the BMD begins to fall (without, of course, any change in external bone size, unless fracture occurs). The fall implies a loss of bone tissue without any change in measured area (or, by implication, volume) and is the result of an imbalance between osteoblastic and osteoclastic activities in favour of resorption. The fall is linear in men but has an accelerated phase in women in the first postmenopausal decade.

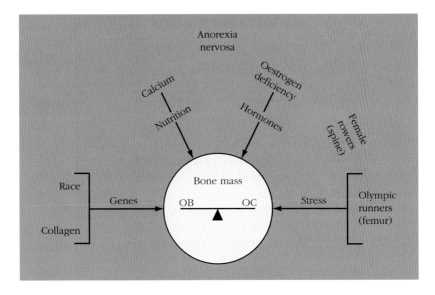

Figure 2.12 *The major determinants of bone mass, with examples. Bone mass is reduced by oestrogen deficiency and malnutrition (anorexia nervosa) and increased by mechanical forces. (OB = osteoblast; OC = osteoclast.)*

Since uncorrected peak BMD in women is lower than that in men, and since there is an accelerated postmenopausal loss, the BMD is lower in women than in men at any adult age and particularly after the menopause. This has important implications for fracture (Chapter 3). However, the sex difference in peak BMD is largely abolished when correction is made for lean body mass; likewise, the peak true volumetric spinal density differs little between men and women.

Low bone mass

The causes of low bone mass occupy much of the following chapters. Most can be understood from the known physiology of bone. The amount of bone in the mature adult depends on the peak bone mass and the subsequent loss. The impact of the genome, and early environment, on the rate of bone gain during growth is the subject of intensive current investigation. Several genetic markers for low peak bone mass have been suggested, and recent observations that weight

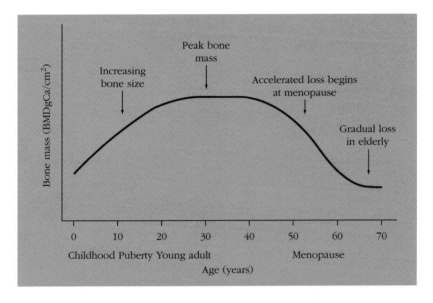

Figure 2.13 *A diagram to show the changes in bone mass (expressed as bone mineral density, BMD) with age in women. (See also Figures 4.8 and 4.11.)*

in infancy is a predictor of adult bone mass suggest that the skeletal growth trajectory might be programmed by gene–environment interactions during intrauterine and early post-natal life. In addition to those factors already discussed, a low peak bone mass may result from endocrine (hypogonadism in both sexes), chromosomal (Turner's syndrome) and nutritional (coeliac disease) factors; peak bone mass is also reduced by certain lifestyle factors, such as smoking, alcoholism and immobility. Excessive bone loss also results from these lifestyle influences, and also, most importantly, an early natural or surgical menopause. These are dealt with in more detail later.

Osteopenia and osteoporosis

Osteoporosis can be defined largely in qualitative terms as a disease characterized by low bone mass and microarchitectural deterioration of bone tissue, leading to enhanced bone fragility and a consequent increase in fracture risk. The increased facilities for accurate and reproducible measurement of bone density and its demonstrated

27

relation to future fracture have made quantitative definitions increasingly relevant. According to a WHO definition osteopenia is said to exist when the bone density (BMD) or bone mineral content (BMC) lies between −1 and −2.5 SD of the young normal mean; osteoporosis exists where the reduction is more than 2.5 SD below the peak bone mass[17,18]. These values in relation to peak bone mass are referred to as a T score; when expressed in relation to age-matched controls, the SD values are known as Z scores. These definitions are discussed in future chapters.

Key points

■ Bone is a metabolically active tissue composed of a mineralized organic bone matrix produced by specialized bone cells. These cells work in teams to remove (osteoclasts) and to replace (osteoblasts) bone tissue. Changes in bone mass depend on the balance between these activities.

■ The strength of bone depends on its structure (cortical and trabecular) and on the integrity of its mineral (hydroxyapatite) and matrix (collagen) components.

■ The activity of bone cells can be assessed by biochemical measurements.

■ The amount of bone and its density varies with age and disease. The main determinants of bone mass are genetic and mechanical factors influenced by endocrine and nutritional status.

References

1 Smith R. Bone in health and disease. In: Maddison PJ, Isenberg DA, Woo P, Glass DN, eds. *Oxford Textbook of Rheumatology.* 2nd Edn. Oxford: Oxford University Press, 1997; 421–440.

2 Noda M. *Cellular and Molecular Biology of Bone.* San Diego: Academic Press, 1993.

3 Raisz LG. Physiology of bone. In: Becker KL, ed. *Principles and Practice of Endocrinology and Metabolism,* 2nd Edn. Philadelphia: Lippincott, 1995; 447–55.

4 Royce PM, Steinmann B. *Connective Tissue and its Heritable Disorders.* New York: Wiley-Liss, 1993.

5 Marcus R, Feldman D, Kelsey J. *Osteoporosis.* New York: Academic Press, 1996.

6 Bilézikian JP, Raisz LG, Rodan GA. *Principles of Bone Biology.* San Diego: Academic Press, 1996.

7 Macdonald BR, Gowen M. The cell biology of bone. *Baillière's Clinical Rheumatology, Vol. 7.,* 1993; 421–443.

8 Smith R. Disorders of the skeleton. In: Weatherall DJ, Ledingham JGG, Warrell DA, eds. *Oxford Textbook of Medicine,* 3rd Edn. Oxford: Oxford University Press, 1995; 3055–95.

9 Hulmes DJS. The collagen super family — diverse structures and assemblies. *Essays Biochem* 1992; **27**: 49–67.

10 Hardingham TE, Fosang AJ. Proteoglycans: many forms and many functions. *FASEB J* 1992; **6**: 861–70.

11 Wozney JM, Bone morphogenetic proteins and their gene expression. In: Noda N, ed. *Cellular and Molecular Biology of Bone.* New York: Academic Press, 1993; 131–67.

12 Manolagas SC, Jilka RL. Bone marrow, cytokines and bone remodelling. *N Eng J Med* 1995; **332**: 305–11.

13 Fraser DR. Vitamin D. *Lancet* 1995; **345** : 104–6.

14 Spector TD, Keen RW, Arden NK, Morrison NA, Major PJ, Nguyen TV, Kelly PJ, Baker JR, Sambrook PN, Lanchbury JS. Influence of vitamin D receptor genotype on bone mineral density in postmenopausal women; a twin study in Britain. *Br Med J* 1995; **310**: 1357–60.

15 Editorial. Pyridinium cross links as markers of bone resorption. *Lancet* 1992; **240**: 278–9.

16 Compston JE, Bone density: BMC, BMD or corrected BMD? *Bone* 1995; **16**: 5–7.

17 Kanis JA, Melton J, Christiansen C, Johnston CC, Khaltaev N. The diagnosis of osteoporosis. *J Bone Miner Res* 1994; **9**: 1137–41.

Chapter 3

Nature and extent of the problem

Introduction

When the term 'osteoporosis' entered medical parlance in France and Germany during the nineteenth century, it implied a histological diagnosis ('porous bone') that was subsequently refined to mean that bone tissue of normal composition, while normally mineralized, was present in reduced quantity. This approach culminates today in attempts to define osteoporosis on the basis of low bone mass, which can be assessed *in vivo* by a variety of non-invasive densitometric techniques. Clinically, however, osteoporosis is recognized by the occurrence of characteristic fractures. Indeed, the realization that these fractures might result from an age-related reduction in bone quality antedated the histological approach to definition. This historical line of thought translates into the view that, to be clinically meaningful, any definition of osteoporosis must include fracture. A study group of the World Health Organization (WHO) has recently attempted a synthesis of these two complementary notions of osteoporosis[1]. This chapter summarizes the epidemiological data concerning the frequency of osteoporosis and the impact that the condition has on society.

Magnitude of the problem

How many people suffer from osteoporosis? It is clear from the Introduction that different answers will be given to this question according to whether osteoporosis is defined on the basis of bone mass alone, or whether fracture is a prerequisite for the disorder.

Bone mass

Implicit in the definition of osteoporosis by bone mass alone is the notion of a relationship between the amount of bone and fracture risk. Low bone mass is therefore analogous to high blood pressure or an elevated serum cholesterol concentration. The risk of fracture increases when bone mass declines, just as the risk of stroke rises with increasing blood pressure and as hypercholesterolaemia leads to an increased risk of myocardial infarction. Data from an age-stratified random sample of women in Rochester, Minnesota, USA[2], were extrapolated to derive the prevalence of osteoporosis in each age group using the WHO definition (see page 28)[1]. As can be seen in Figure 3.1, most White women under the age of 50 years have normal bone density at all four skeletal sites, and osteoporosis is rare. With advancing age, however, a greater proportion has osteopenia or osteoporosis (Table 3.1). Among women aged 80 years and over, for example, 32% have osteoporosis of the lumbar spine, 47.5% of the hip and 70% at any of the hip, spine or radius. Of the latter group, 60% have experienced one or more fractures of the proximal femur, vertebra, distal forearm, proximal humerus, or pelvis. Overall, an estimated 16.8 million (54%) of postmenopausal white women in the United States have osteopenia and another 9.4 million (30%) have osteoporosis. About 4.8 million women (51% of the osteoporotic women and 16% of all White women age 50 years or above) are estimated to have established osteoporosis, i.e. osteoporosis with fracture[3]. The latter figure is probably an underestimate since most fractures in elderly women are related at least in part to low bone mass, but only selected fracture sites were considered here. Estimates from other parts of the world are currently being assembled, but hip bone density data from the United Kingdom

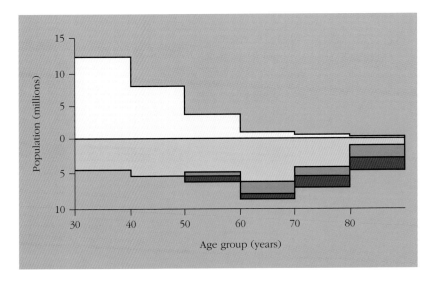

Figure 3.1 Estimated skeletal status of White women in the USA, 1990, by age group. Osteopenia is bone density of the hip, spine or distal forearm > 1.0 but ≤ 2.5 SD below the young normal mean; osteoporosis is bone density at one or more of these sites > 2.5 SD below the mean. ■ Established osteoporosis, i.e., with fracture; ▨ osteoporosis; ▥ osteopenia; □ normal. (Reproduced from ref. 2, with permission.)

suggest that about 23% of women aged 50 years and above have osteoporosis according to the WHO definition[1]. This proportion would rise considerably if other sites (such as the spine and forearm) were included.

Fracture

Osteoporotic fractures share three distinctive features: incidence rates that are greater among women than men, rates that increase steeply with age, and a predilection for skeletal sites containing a large proportion of trabecular bone. Fractures of the hip, spine and distal forearm share these characteristics and are the sites most frequently affected in osteoporotic individuals. Fractures of the proximal humerus and distal femur also reveal these epidemiological characteristics. The advent of bone densitometry has permitted the relationship between bone mass and fracture risk to be evaluated

Table 3.1 Proportion of Rochester, Minnesota, USA, women with bone mineral measurements more than 2.5 SD below the mean for young normal women

Age group (years)	Lumbar spine (%)	Either hip (%)	Mid-radius (%)	Spine, hip or mid-radius (%)
50–59	7.6	3.9	3.7	14.8
60–69	11.8	8.0	11.8	21.6
70–79	25.0	24.5	23.1	38.5
≥80	32.0	47.5	50.0	70.0
Total[†]	16.5	16.2	17.4	30.3

[†]Age adjusted to the population structure of 1990 US White women ≥50 years of age. (From ref. 2, with permission.)

directly, and it is now recognised that other types of fractures in the elderly for example, those of the hand, foot, rib and clavicle, are also associated with low bone density.

There are few data regarding the lifetime risk of osteoporotic fractures. Using fracture incidence rates from the USA (which are around 25% greater than those in Great Britain), the estimated lifetime risk of a hip fracture is 17.5% in 50-year-old White women and 6.0% in 50-year-old White men (Table 3.2)[3]. This contrasts with risks of 15.6 and 5.0% for clinically diagnosed vertebral fractures, and 16 and 2.5% for distal forearm fractures, in White women and men, respectively. The lifetime risk of any of the three fractures is 39.7% for women and 13.1% for men from age 50 years onward (Table 3.2).

Table 3.2 Lifetime fracture risk in 50-year-old White men and women*

Fracture site	Lifetime risk	
	Men (%)	Women (%)
Hip fracture	6.0	17.5
Clinically diagnosed vertebral fracture	5.0	15.6
Distal forearm fracture	2.5	16.0
Any of the above	13.1	39.7

*Residents of Rochester, Minnesota, USA.
(From ref. 3, with permission.)

Fracture epidemiology

Fracture incidence in the community is bimodal, with peaks in youth and in the very elderly. In young people, fractures of the long bones predominate, often following substantial trauma, and the incidence is greater in young men than in young women. Above the age of 35 years, overall fracture incidence in women climbs steeply, so that female rates become twice those in men. At least 1.3 million fractures in the USA each year have been attributed to osteoporosis, presuming that 70% of all fractures in persons aged 45 years or over are due to low bone mass[4]. The three sites most closely associated with osteoporosis are the hip, spine and distal forearm. However, the epidemiologic characteristics of these three types of fracture differ (Figure 3.2), suggesting different causes[5].

Hip fracture

Hip fractures may involve the subcapital, trans-cervical, inter- and sub-trochanteric regions of the proximal femur. Hip fracture is the most

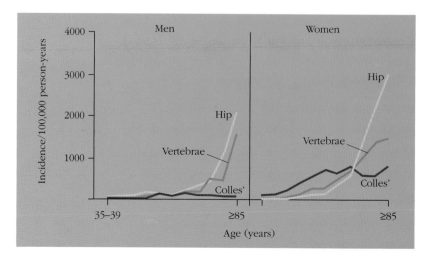

Figure 3.2 *Age-specific incidence rates for hip, vertebral and distal forearm fractures in men and women. Data derived from the population of Rochester, Minnesota, USA (Reproduced from ref. 5, with permission.)*

severe osteoporotic fracture. Most follow a fall from the standing position, although they are known to occur spontaneously. Overall, 90% of hip fractures occur among people aged 50 years and over, and 80% occur in women. The average age at which hip fractures occur in Great Britain is 79 years.

Hip fractures are seasonal, occurring more frequently during winter in temperate countries, but the majority follow falls indoors and are not related to slipping on icy pavements. This seasonal variation in hip fracture is as marked in the southern hemisphere as it is in Europe and North America. Proposed explanations include abnormal neuromuscular function at lower temperatures, and a winter time reduction in sunlight exposure.

Age- and sex-adjusted hip fracture rates are generally higher in White than in Black or Asian populations, although urbanization in certain parts of Africa may have led to recent increases in hip fracture rates. Furthermore, the pronounced female preponderance observed in White populations is not seen among Blacks or Asians, in whom male and female rates are similar.

Geographic variation in hip fracture has been studied extensively in the USA, Sweden and the UK. In the USA, there is a North–South gradient with highest rates of fracture in the south east. Other factors that seem deleterious include socioeconomic deprivation, decreased sunlight exposure and fluoridated water supply. Living in a rural community appears to be a protective factor in Sweden and the UK (East Anglia).

Demographic changes (changes in age structure of the population) over the next 60 years will lead to huge increases in the number of hip fractures requiring medical care. In Europe, the growth of the elderly fraction of the population will increase fracture numbers by 80% by the year 2025. This increase will be even more dramatic in Asia. Superimposed on these changes in population age structure are time trends in the age-specific incidence of hip fracture, which has been observed to increase in recent decades. However, the most recent data show a slowing of this increase.

Vertebral fracture

Epidemiological information on vertebral fractures has been hampered by the absence of a universally accepted definition of vertebral deformity from lateral thoracolumbar radiographs, and because a substantial proportion of vertebral deformities are asymptomatic. The application of recently developed definitions to various population samples in the USA has permitted estimation of the incidence of new vertebral fractures in the general population[6]. The incidence of all vertebral deformities among postmenopausal White women has been estimated to be around three times that of hip fracture. However, the incidence of clinically ascertained vertebral deformities is around 30% of this total figure. The overall age-adjusted female to male incidence ratio for these deformities is 1.9. The most frequent vertebral levels involved are T8, T12 and L1, the weakest regions in the spine (Figure 3.3). Vertebral fracture rarely leads to hospitalization in the UK: as few as 2%

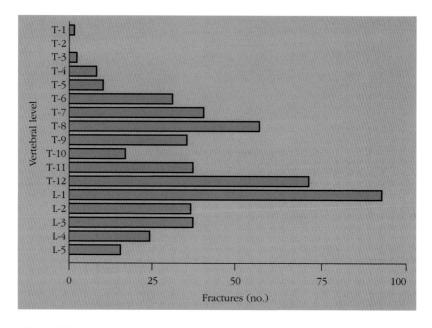

Figure 3.3 *Anatomical level of vertebral fracture in 341 Rochester, Minnesota, men and women with clinically diagnosed vertebral fractures. (Derived from ref. 6 with permission.)*

of patients may be admitted. Clinical coding inadequacies may underestimate this figure. Its economic burden is mainly due to outpatient care, provision of nursing care and lost working days; in addition, of those patients seeking medical attention, at least 80% had a detectable deformity. In women, fracture is associated with only minor or moderate trauma (90%), whereas in men 37% of fractures may be associated with significant injury.

The results of a large, population-based survey of 14,000 men and women throughout Europe have shed much light on the epidemiology of vertebral fractures[7]. The overall prevalence was around 12% in both sexes, but there was a much steeper increase in frequency with age among women. Vertebral deformities were significantly associated with back pain and height loss in both sexes.

Wrist fracture

Wrist fractures display a different pattern of occurrence from hip or spine fractures[8]. In White women, rates increase linearly between 40 and 65 years of age and then stabilize. In men, the incidence remains constant between 20 and 80 years. The reason for the plateau in female incidence remains obscure, but may relate to a change in the pattern of falling with advancing age. As in the case of hip fracture, most wrist fractures occur in women and around one-half occur among women aged 65 years and over. The winter peak in wrist fracture incidence is even greater than that seen for hip fracture.

Impact of osteoporotic fractures

The adverse outcomes of osteoporotic fractures fall into three broad categories; namely mortality, morbidity and cost (Table 3.3).

Mortality

The influence of hip, spine and distal forearm fractures on survival is only beginning to be recognized, and appears to differ with the type

Table 3.3 The impact of osteoporotic fractures in British women

	Hip	Vertebral*	Forearm
Mortality[†]	0.83	0.82	1.00
Morbidity			
Lifetime risk (%)	14	11	13
Cases/year	60,000	40,000	50,000
Disability	+++	++	+

Annual estimated cost   All sites combined = UK £942 × 10[6]

*Clinically diagnosed vertebral fractures.
[†]Relative survival (proportion surviving compared with an age-matched non-fracture cohort) at 5 years following diagnosis.

of fracture (Figure 3.4). Hip fractures lead to an overall reduction in survival of 17% at 5 years. The majority of excess deaths occur within the first 3 months after the fracture and diminish with time so that, after 3 months or so, survival is comparable to that of similar-aged men and women in the general population. Mortality differs, however, by age and sex. In one population-based study[9], a relative survival of

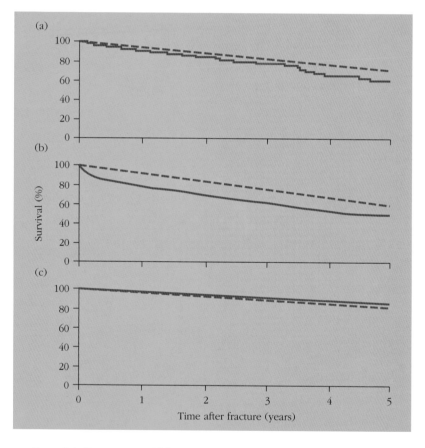

Figure 3.4 *Five-year survival following diagnosis of (a) vertebral, (b) hip or (c) distal forearm fracture. Figures show observed survival (———) for a fracture cohort from Rochester, Minnesota, and expected data (– – – –) for individuals of like age and sex. (Reproduced from ref. 9, with permission.)*

92% was found for White hip fracture victims under 75 years of age, compared with only 83% for those aged 75 years and over at the time of fracture. Despite their greater age at the time of fracture, survival was better among women than men in this study. The sex difference has been observed in hospital-based studies as well, and appears to arise from the greater frequency of other chronic diseases among men who sustain hip fractures. Most deaths following hip fracture are probably unrelated to falling *per se*, even though accidental falls are among the leading causes of death among the elderly of Western nations. Some deaths are attributable to acute complications of the fracture, or of its surgical management. However, most appear to be due to serious coexisting illnesses.

Until recently it was assumed that osteoporotic vertebral fractures were not attended by significant mortality. However, population-based data relating to clinically diagnosed vertebral fractures now show that overall survival among patients is substantially worse than expected[8]. At 5 years following fracture diagnosis, the estimated survival was 61% compared with an expected survival for those of like age and sex of 76% (giving a relative survival of 0.82). The proportionate excess of deaths following those vertebral fractures that reach clinical attention is thus comparable to that following hip fracture (Table 3.4). In marked contrast, there does not appear to be any excess mortality among patients who sustain distal forearm fractures.

The reason for the excess death rate following vertebral fracture is not clear. Examination of the underlying causes of death in this cohort of 335 men and women revealed no cause-specific associations. Furthermore, there was no evidence of the early excess seen following hip fracture, suggesting that the impaired survival following vertebral fracture does not result from the injury *per se* but is due instead to an indirect association with comorbid conditions that lead to an increased risk of osteoporosis. This explanation would accord with the observation that low bone density is itself associated with excess mortality from various non-skeletal causes.

Table 3.4 Relative survival following vertebral, hip and distal forearm fractures among residents of Rochester, Minnesota, according to duration of follow-up from diagnosis

Time from diagnosis (years)	Relative survival*		
	Vertebral	Hip	Forearm
1	0.96 (0.92–0.99)	0.88 (0.85–0.91)	1.00 (0.98–1.02)
2	0.93 (0.87–0.99)	0.87 (0.83–0.90)	1.00 (0.97–1.03)
3	0.92 (0.86–0.98)	0.86 (0.82–0.90)	1.01 (0.98–1.04)
4	0.84 (0.75–0.92)	0.83 (0.78–0.88)	0.99 (0.95–1.04)
5	0.82 (0.71–0.93)	0.83 (0.77–0.89)	1.00 (0.95–1.05)

*95% confidence intervals in parentheses.

Morbidity

The morbidity associated with osteoporotic fractures is difficult to assess because the prevalence of disability and the incidence of fractures both rise steeply with age. However, it has been estimated (after allowing for the functional impairment expected in similarly aged people) that fractures of the hip, spine and distal forearm result in 6.7% of all women becoming dependent in the basic activities of daily living, and cause nursing home care in a further 7.8% for an average of 7.6 years.

As with mortality, hip fractures contribute most to this disability and service utilization. Patients with hip fractures almost invariably require admission to hospital; in 1985, the average length of hospital stay in England and Wales was 30 days. Thus 3500 National Health Service hospital beds are used in the management of this condition daily. While these patients are at high risk of developing acute complications, the most important long-term outcome is impairment of the ability to walk. Around 20% of patients are unable to walk even before the fracture but, of those who had been able to walk, half cannot walk independently afterwards. Ultimately, up to one-third of hip fracture victims may become totally dependent, and many will require prolonged care in institutions (Tables 3.5 and 3.6).

The health impact of vertebral fractures has proved considerably more difficult to quantify. As stated earlier, only a minority of new vertebral deformities come to clinical attention. None the less, vertebral fractures in patients aged 45 years and older account for about 52,000 hospital admissions in the USA and 2188 in England and Wales each year. The major clinical consequences of vertebral fracture are back pain, kyphosis and height loss. New compression fractures may give rise to severe back pain, which typically decreases in severity over several weeks or months.

Table 3.5 Disability following hip fracture (1 year)

Activity	Percentage unable
Independent walking	40
One ADL (dressing/washing)	60
One IADL (shopping/driving)	80

ADL=activity of daily living; IADL=independent activity of daily living.

Table 3.6 Social consequences of hip fracture (1 year)

Event	Probability (%)
Hospitalization	100
Nursing home < 1 year	27
Nursing home > 1 year	14
Home support	30

This pain is associated with exquisite localized tenderness and paravertebral muscle spasm that markedly limits spinal movements.

A more protracted clinical course affects a proportion of patients, who have a history of chronic pain experienced while standing and during physical stress, particularly bending. In one treatment study, for example, patients were noted to have persistent pain for 6 months following fracture. This chronic pain is thought to arise from spinal extensor muscle weakness, as well as the altered spinal biomechanics that result from vertebral deformation. A number of indices of physical function, self-esteem, body image and mood also appear to be adversely affected in patients with vertebral fractures. Whenever self-report scales of functional status or quality of life have been applied to patients with vertebral fractures, scores are found to be worse for those with more severe or multiple deformities.

Despite the fact that only around one-fifth of all patients with distal forearm fractures are hospitalized, they account for some 50,000 hospital admissions and over 400,000 physician visits in the USA each year, and 10,000 hospital admissions in Great Britain. Admission rates vary markedly with age, such that only 16% of the forearm fractures occurring in women aged 45–54 years required inpatient care, compared with 76% of those in women aged 85 years and over. There is up to a 30% risk of algodystrophy after these fractures, as well as an increased likelihood of neuropathies and post-traumatic arthritis. Nearly one-half of all patients report only fair or poor functional outcomes at 6 months following distal forearm fracture.

Costs of fractures

The total cost of osteoporosis is difficult to assess because it includes inpatient and outpatient medical care, loss of working days and chronic nursing home costs. The direct hospital costs of osteoporosis stem mainly from management of patients with hip fractures. These were recently estimated at £160 million annually, and comprise 71% of the annual direct inpatient hospital cost for all fractures of £226 million. This compares with a figure of $2.8 billion in the USA. When outpatient costs were added to this US estimate, the total direct cost of osteoporosis came to $5.2 billion for women alone. An estimated total annual cost in the UK population is £942 million.

Future projections

The financial and health-related costs of osteoporosis can only rise in future generations. Life expectancy is increasing around the globe and the number of elderly individuals is rising in every geographic region. There are currently about 323 million individuals aged 65 years or over, and this number is expected to reach 1555 million by the year 2050[9]. The demographic changes alone can be expected to cause the number of hip fractures occurring among people aged 35 years and over throughout the world to increase from 1.66 million in 1990, to 6.26 million in 2050 (Figure 3.5). Using current estimates for hip fracture incidence from various parts of the world, it can be calculated that around one-half of all hip fractures to occur among elderly people in 1990 take place in Europe and North America. By 2050, the rapid ageing of the Asian and Latin American populations will result in the European and North American contribution falling to only 25%, with over one-half of all fractures occurring in Asia. It is clear, therefore, that osteoporosis will become a truly global problem over the next half century, and that measures are urgently required to halt the progress of this trend.

There are also trends in fracture incidence independent of age[10]. These trends have been best studied for hip fracture. Figure 3.6 depicts the age-adjusted changes in hip fracture incidence (derived using national hospital discharge statistics) among men and women in England and Wales during the period 1968–1985. It shows a linear increase in rates, occurring in both sexes, until around 1978, with a plateau in rates thereafter. Similar time trends have been reported from many Western nations, but the times at which rates level off seem to differ. Thus, among women in the northern USA, rates increased between 1935 and 1960 but have remained stable since. In other European countries, increases are still being observed.

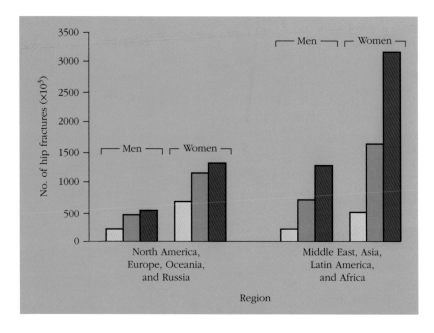

Figure 3.5 *Projections for numbers of hip fractures worldwide in 1990* □*, 2025* ▣ *and 2050* ■*. (Derived from ref. 10, with permission.)*

There are three broad explanations for these trends. First, they might represent some increasingly prevalent current risk factor for osteoporosis or falling. Time trends for a number of such risk factors, including oophorectomy, oestrogen replacement therapy, cigarette smoking, alcohol consumption and dietary calcium intake, do not match those observed for hip fractures. Physical activity, however, appears to be a likely candidate. There is ample epidemiological evidence linking inactivity to the risk of hip fracture, whether this effect is mediated through bone density, the risk of falls, or both. Furthermore, some of the steepest secular trends have been observed in Asian countries such as Hong Kong, which have witnessed dramatic reductions in the customary activity levels of their populations in recent decades.

The second explanation for the time trend is that the elderly population is becoming increasingly frail. The prevalence of disability

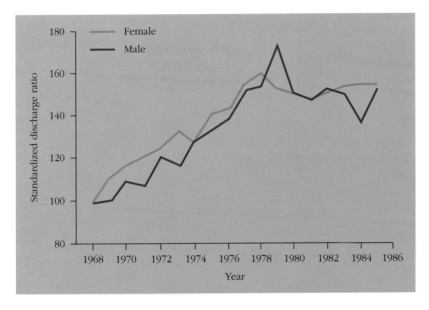

Figure 3.6 *Age-standardized changes in hospital discharge rates for hip fracture in England and Wales, 1968–1985. Changes are expressed relative to the rate in each sex for 1968. (Reproduced from ref. 11, with permission.)*

is known to rise with age, and to be greater among women at any age than among men. As many of the contributory disorders to this frailty are independently associated with osteoporosis and the risk of falling, this tendency might have contributed to the increases in Western nations during earlier decades of this century.

Finally, the trends could arise from a cohort phenomenon — some adverse influence on bone mass or the risk of falling that acted at an earlier time but is now manifesting as a rising incidence in successive generations of the elderly. Differences between succeeding generations explain some of the trends in adult height during this century; similar effects on the skeleton are likely.

Incidence rates for fractures at other skeletal sites have also risen during the last half of the twentieth century. Studies from Malmo in southern Sweden have suggested age-specific increases for distal forearm, ankle, proximal humeral and vertebral fractures. In many instances, these trends appeared in men as well as women. The observation for vertebral fractures is particularly important as it points to a changing prevalence of osteoporosis, rather than falling, as a general explanation for these trends. Recent data from the northern USA have confirmed increases in the incidence of clinically diagnosed vertebral fractures among postmenopausal women until the early 1960s, with a plateau in rates thereafter. As with the Swedish data, these rate changes paralleled those observed for hip fractures in the same population.

Fracture incidence in general practice
Tables 3.7–3.9 show the burden of osteoporotic fractures that would be encountered in a typical British general practice of 2000 people, on the basis of the epidemiological data outlined above.

Table 3.7 Incidence of osteoporotic fractures in an average general practice

Type	No./year
◾ All fractures	7–8
◾ Hip fractures	2–3
◾ Wrist fractures	2
◾ Vertebral fracture	
Clinical	2
Deformity	5

Table 3.8 Prevalence of vertebral deformity in an average general practice

Age (years)	Men (n)	Women (n)
45–54	2	4
55–64	4	6
65–74	7	11
75–84	12	20
85+	4	7
All	29	48

Table 3.9 Prevalence of osteoporosis* in an average general practice

Age (years)	Men		Women	
	(%)	(n)	(%)	(n)
45–54	1	1	5	6
55–64	5	5	9	9
65–74	5	5	24	23
75–84	17	7	48	33
85+	29	2	61	15
All	6	20	23	86

*Data based on femoral neck bone mass measurements in men and women in UK; osteoporosis defined by the WHO criteria.

The table shows the number of subjects and proportion in each age group.

Key points

■ Osteoporosis is a complex multifactorial disorder in which a variety of pathophysiological mechanisms lead to a progressive reduction in bone strength and an increased risk of fracture.

■ Whether defined by low bone mass or by the occurrence of specific fractures, osteoporosis is clearly a common condition.

■ Of White US women, aged ≥50 years, 54% have low bone mass in the lumbar spine, proximal femur or mid-radius, and 30% are osteoporotic.

■ The estimated lifetime risk of a hip, spine or forearm fracture from the age of 50 years is 39.7% among women and 13.1% among men.

■ This health burden will increase dramatically in future decades.

References

1 Kanis JA and the WHO Study Group. Assessment of fracture risk and its application to screening for postmenopausal osteoporosis: synopsis of a WHO report. *Osteoporosis Int* 1994; **4**: 368–81.

2 Melton LJ. How many women have osteoporosis now? *J Bone Miner Res* 1995; **10**: 175–7.

3 Melton LJ III, Chrischilles EA, Cooper C, Lane AW, Riggs BL. How many women have osteoporosis? *J Bone Miner Res* 1992; **7**: 1005–10.

4 Melton LJ III. Epidemiology of fractures. In: Riggs BL, Melton LJ III, eds. *Osteoporosis: Etiology, Diagnosis, and Management.* New York: Raven Press, 1988; 133–54.

5 Cooper C, Melton LJ. Epidemiology of osteoporosis. *Trends Endocrinol Metab* 1992; **3**: 224–9.

6 Cooper EJ, Atkinson SJ, O'Fallon WM, Melton LJ III. The incidence of clinically diagnosed vertebral fractures: a population-based study in Rochester, Minnesota, 1985–1989. *J Bone Miner Res* 1992; **7**: 221–7.

7 O'Neill TW, Felsenberg D, Varlow J *et al.* The prevalence of vertebral deformity in European men and women: the European Vertebral Osteoporosis Study. *J Bone Miner Res* 1996; **11**: 1010–18.

8 Owen RA, Melton LJ III, Johnson KA, Ilstrup DM, Riggs BL. Incidence of Colles' fracture in a North American community. *Am J Public Health* 1982; **72**: 605–7.

9 Cooper C, Atkinson EJ, Jacobsen SJ, O'Fallon WM, Melton LJ III. Population-based study of survival after osteoporotic fractures. *Am J Epidemiol* 1993; **137**: 1001–5.

10 Cooper EJ, Campion G, Melton LJ III. Hip fractures in the elderly: a worldwide projection. *Osteoporosis Int* 1992; **2**: 285–9.

11 Spector C, Cooper EJ, Lewis AF. Trends in admissions for hip fracture in England and Wales, 1968–85. *Br Med J* 1990; **300**: 1173–4.

Chapter 4

Clinical recognition and diagnosis of osteoporosis

Introduction

Over the last 30 years significant progress has been made in the development of methods of non-invasive assessment of bone mass and, with it, an increasing understanding of the patterns of bone loss that occur in health and disease. Treatment options now exist, not only to arrest bone loss but also to restore bone mass. This has increased the importance of timely diagnosis and risk assessment in order to identify patients who are most likely to benefit from treatments currently available.

A fundamental prerequisite to making a diagnosis of osteoporosis is awareness of the condition in the mind of the physician. Consideration of osteoporosis as a possibility in differential diagnosis is required by general practitioners and specialists, allied professionals in nursing, physiotherapy and occupational therapy, and all those involved in the care of the elderly (see Chapter 8). Today's health professionals have rarely received much undergraduate or postgraduate education on the subject of osteoporosis. It is the comparative ignorance of this condition and the fact that it lies, as a subject, between many of the specialities, that is a major barrier to its recognition and management.

Definition of osteoporosis

The currently accepted conceptual definition of osteoporosis is of a systemic skeletal disease characterized by low bone mass and microarchitectural deterioration of bone tissue, with a consequent increase in bone fragility and susceptibility to fracture risk[1]. This definition of osteoporosis captures the notion that BMD is an important component of fracture risk, but that other abnormalities, both skeletal and extra-skeletal, also contribute. However, BMD can be measured with a precision and accuracy greater than other skeletal and extra-skeletal factors, and its measurement forms the basis for the diagnosis of osteoporosis. The relationship between BMD and fracture risk is continuous. An estimate of bone mineral provides an effective estimate of fracture risk in the same way that blood pressure predicts the risk of stroke. It is possible, therefore, to choose an arbitrary value for BMD which constitutes a threshold below which fracture risk is unacceptably high. Fracture thresholds may be derived from the range of density measurements made in a population with osteoporotic fractures, or from their distribution in the young healthy adult population.

For diagnostic purposes, a threshold of BMD has been proposed by the World Health Organization (WHO) for Caucasian women, based on the distribution of skeletal mass in young healthy individuals. There is a normal distribution of bone mineral in young healthy women (peak bone mass) irrespective of the measurement method used, so bone density values in individuals are often expressed in standard deviation (SD) units in relation to a reference population. This reduces the problem associated with differences in calibration between instruments. When SDs are used in relation to the young healthy population, this is referred to as the T-score, where the mean is ascribed a value of zero. According to the WHO definition, *osteoporosis* is defined as a value more than 2.5 SD below the young normal adult mean. *Severe/established osteoporosis* refers to individuals with osteoporosis who have sustained a fragility fracture in addition. *Osteopenia* refers to individuals with values between 1 and 2.5 SD below the young adult mean[2].

Types of osteoporosis

Osteoporosis may be the end result of a number of pathological processes (Table 4.1). Bone loss commences in both men and women during the fourth decade of life. There are two principal reasons for this bone loss:

■ progressive decline in the responsiveness of the osteoblast to mechanical stimuli, and

■ a gradual reduction in the efficiency of calcium absorption which results in secondary hyperparathyroidism and increased osteoclastic bone resorption.

Superimposed on the age-related change in bone mass among women is the influence of oestrogen deficiency following the menopause. Although age-related and postmenopausal bone loss are the most frequent causes of osteoporosis, a number of secondary causes have been established which are outlined below. These are important, because they are sometimes reversible. The outline in Table 4.1 is not intended to be a comprehensive description of secondary causes, but to be an *aide-mémoire* of those most frequently seen in clinical practice.

Secondary types of osteoporosis

Corticosteroid excess in Cushing's syndrome is recognized by the appearance of striae, muscle wasting and proximal myopathy, with hypertension and glycosuria; it is often iatrogenic in patients taking corticosteroid treatment for disorders such as rheumatoid arthritis, systemic lupus erythematosis, polymyalgia rheumatica, temporal arteritis or asthma. Osteoporosis results mainly from the suppression of osteoblast function. The resulting fractures are often painless and heal with a large amount of callus.

The skeleton's response to the administration of exogenous corticosteroid is very variable, but, in some cases, considerable bone may be lost in the first few months of treatment.

Table 4.1 Types of osteoporosis

Primary/idiopathic
- Age-related
- Postmenopausal

Secondary causes
- Endocrine
  - Cushing's syndrome
  - Thyrotoxicosis
  - Hypogonadism (primary or secondary)
  - Pituitary insufficiency
  - Athletic amenorrhoea
- Drugs
  - Corticosteroids
  - Long-term heparin use
  - Anticonvulsant use
  - Cytotoxic agents
- Inherited
  - Turner's syndrome
  - Osteogenesis imperfecta
  - Homocystinuria
- Nutritional
  - Anorexia nervosa
  - Alcoholism
  - Malabsorption syndromes
- Immobility
  - General (e.g. lack of weight-bearing exercise)
  - Local (e.g. rheumatoid arthritis, hemiplegia, fracture)
- Other (rare)
  - Chronic hepatic disease
  - Juvenile
  - Pregnancy
  - Mastocytosis

Thyroxine excess, when prolonged, results in increased bone turnover with resorption in excess of formation. Hypercalcaemia with raised inorganic phosphate and alkaline phosphatase levels may occur.

Oestrogen deficiency (other than postmenopausal) may result from premature ovarian failure. Excessive exercise may also lead to a disturbance of ovarian function.

Androgen deficiency in men resulting from hypogonadism is not common. Clinical features include the absence of secondary sexual characteristics, with a smooth skin, a high-pitched voice, low hairline and skeletal disproportion (long limbs relative to the trunk).

Hypopituitarism leads to the failure of other endocrine systems. In children this results in infantilism, with a combination of short stature and hypogonadism. Pituitary failure in the adult is usually the result of a pituitary tumour and is a rare cause of osteoporosis. Confusingly, the X-ray appearance of the skeleton in acromegaly resulting from pituitary overactivity is sometimes referred to as osteoporotic.

Inherited factors clearly influence bone mass. In addition, osteoporosis occurs in specific chromosomal defects such as Turner's syndrome (XO) and Kleinfelter's syndrome (XXY); in both cases, sex hormone deficiency is an important factor. In osteogenesis imperfecta there is mutation in the gene for type I collagen (the main collagen of bone, Chapter 2). In the mild (type 1) form there is a 50% reduction in type I collagen which leads to a reduced BMD and increased susceptibility to fractures from childhood onwards. In most cases there is a dominant family history, and clinical findings include blue sclera, dentinogenesis imperfecta, hypermobility and early onset deafness.

Nutritional causes of bone loss include malnutrition (in its broadest sense) and malabsorption. Patients with coeliac disease have a lower bone density than normal. In the Western world, anorexia nervosa represents an important cause of malnutrition; the associated low bone density probably results also from oestrogen deficiency secondary to starvation.

Idiopathic juvenile osteoporosis may rarely occur in childhood. The condition is often self-limiting; improvement often begins towards the end of adolescence as the rate of growth slows. The cause is unknown but it is important to exclude leukaemia, which may present with similar skeletal changes.

Pregnancy-associated osteoporosis usually presents in the third trimester of the first pregnancy, with back pain resulting from vertebral fracture. The condition improves rapidly after delivery and recurrence in subsequent pregnancies is unusual. The cause is unknown.

Clinical evaluation

History

Osteoporosis is most frequently diagnosed following a low trauma fracture (Figure 4.1). The occurrence of hip and forearm fractures is generally easy to identify in the history, whereas vertebral fractures may remain clinically silent. Loss of height, the presence of back pain and a progressive kyphosis leading to a so called Dowager's hump (Figure 4.2) are the most frequent presenting features of vertebral fracture. Since patients may not recognize their own loss of height, questioning of relatives may be helpful. Clothes that previously fitted may no longer do so, despite insignificant weight change.

Epidemiological studies suggest that around 40% of patients with vertebral deformities report previous back pain. However, back pain is a very frequent presenting complaint in primary care and is most often due to soft tissue lesions, intervertebral disc prolapse and

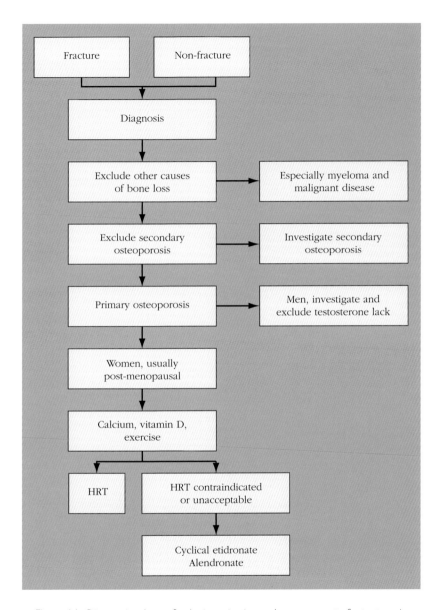

Figure 4.1 *Diagnostic scheme for the investigation and management of osteoporosis. (Reproduced from Smith R. Investigation of osteoporosis. Clinical Endocrinology 1996; 44: 371–4, with permission.)*

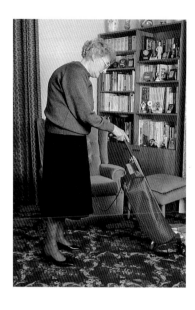

Figure 4.2 *Dowager's hump.*
The figure demonstrates the
thoracic kyphosis due to
vertebral collapse in an elderly
woman.

osteoarthritis of the facet joints. Recognition of cases related to osteoporotic collapse therefore requires a high index of suspicion among patients with additional risk factors. Mid-thoracic pain is more likely to represent significant disease than is lumbar pain. Some common causes of back pain are listed in Table 4.2.

In women, a menstrual history should include age of the menarche and menopause, cycle abnormalities during the menstrual years (including any significant periods of amenorrhoea), number of pregnancies, and any gynaecological surgery.

Drug inquiry should include past or present corticosteroid use, anticonvulsant therapy and, in women, details of HRT. Use of bisphosphonates, fluoride, calcitonin and calcium and vitamin D supplements should be ascertained.

To date, there is little evidence to suggest that long-term oral contraceptive use affects bone mineral density. Enquiry about lifestyle factors such as smoking, alcohol excess, exercise and diet is necessary. A dietary history should include any episodes of severe weight loss, especially when associated with bulimia or anorexia.

Table 4.2 Common causes of back pain

Clinical description	*Some causes*
▉ Mechanical — pain affected by movement, and worse on prolonged sitting or standing. Often chronic and relatively mild	Spondylosis Apophyseal osteoarthritis Vertebral hyperostosis Spondylolisthesis Congenital and other structural anomalies Idiopathic
▉ Inflammatory — associated with morning stiffness, often relieved by exercise	Ankylosing spondylitis Other 'spondyloarthropathies' Spondylosis and osteoarthritis
▉ Neurological — impulse pain, root radiation and/or neurological signs	Disc prolapse Spinal stenosis
▉ Sinister — clues may include ill-health, systemic signs and symptoms, isolated areas of severe tenderness, weight loss and fever	Infection — tuberculous, staphylococcal, *Brucella* and others Neoplasia — primary or secondary deposits; myeloma
▉ Metabolic bone disease	
▉ Referred — pain radiating to the back from another source	Numerous thoracic and abdominal causes, e.g. posterior erosion of peptic ulcer
▉ Unclassified — very common	Numerous structural and psychogenic causes

Current and past dietary habits should be explored, with particular reference to foods containing calcium and vitamin D (principally dairy products in a Western diet). Such enquiry should be specific to ethnic groups with different dietary habits. This is particularly important in Asian women in temperate climates — a population at increased risk of vitamin D deficiency.

Inherited factors strongly influence bone density and therefore it is important to recognize close family members who may have or have had osteoporosis. This is most easily obtained by enquiry into fractures and loss of height.

Physical examination

Physical examination requires full assessment of the thoracolumbar spine and measurement of proportions. In young adults, span is approximately equal to height, and crown to pubis length equals pubis to heel. With progressive spinal fractures, an increased thoracic kyphosis may develop ('dowager's hump'; Figure 4.2). This may be accompanied by protrusion of the manubrium sterni and development of a transverse abdominal crease. Many spinal fractures are painless; localized tenderness to pressure may suggest a recent vertebral fracture.

Special investigations

Haematology and biochemistry

Initial laboratory assessments should identify secondary causes of osteoporosis and exclude other disease (such as multiple myeloma or neoplastic bone disease). They should be applied selectively to those for whom clinical suspicion of an underlying disorder exists, and should include the following:

- full blood count: evidence of marrow disturbance (e.g. myeloma) or malabsorptive states (e.g. macrocytosis)
- erythrocyte sedimentation rate (ESR): evidence of underlying chronic inflammatory or malignant disease
- biochemical profile: evidence of severe renal disease or disorders of calcium and phosphate metabolism

- protein electrophoresis and urinary Bence-Jones proteins if myeloma is suspected (ESR elevated)
- so-called liver function tests (including serum albumin): evidence of chronic liver disease (although a raised alkaline phosphatase may suggest Paget's disease), and
- thyroid function tests.

In women with menstrual disturbance or who may be perimenopausal, measurement of serum follicle-stimulating hormone (FSH) and oestradiol may be useful to define ovarian failure. In men with osteoporosis, the serum testosterone concentration, sex-hormone-binding globulin and free-androgen index should be measured.

Recently, there has been considerable interest in the biochemical assessment of bone turnover, particularly in the use of urinary collagen-derived crosslinked peptides as indicators of bone resorption[3]. Other urinary markers of bone resorption are the excretion of calcium, hydroxyproline, hydroxylysine and its glycosides; plasma markers of bone formation are total and bone-specific alkaline phosphatase, osteocalcin and procollagen extension peptides. In addition, plasma tartrate-resistant acid phosphatase derived from osteoclasts may indicate the rate of bone turnover.

During the formation of collagen, the extension peptides are removed from the procollagen molecule shortly after its export from the cell (Chapter 2). These can be measured in plasma and identified according to which end of the procollagen molecule they are derived from (carboxy- or amino-terminal). When the collagen fibres are formed, trifunctional crosslinks involving lysine and hydroxylysine residues and their aldehydes form between the helical part of one molecule and the telopeptide part of another. When collagen fibres are broken down (during bone resorption), peptides containing these crosslinks are excreted in the urine. Although they differ according to their origin and type of crosslink, those pyridinum crosslinks provide a sensitive indicator of bone resorption, independent of dietary collagen. Initial methods of assay used HPLC, but recent commercial kits utilise immunological assays and measure different peptides.

Further development will be necessary before these methods can be useful in routine clinical practice.

Radiology

Thoracolumbar spine X-ray: Radiological investigations are useful to establish the presence or absence of fracture. Clinicians should, however, be mindful of the potential risk of ionizing radiation, which is probably inversely proportional to the age of the subject. Lumbar and thoracic anterior and lateral views (four films) carry an exposure dose of 2.4 MSv, which is equivalent to 120 chest X-rays or 14 months of normal background radiation.

Axial sites have a greater proportion of trabecular to cortical bone than appendicular sites. Spinal vertebral deformity may therefore be the first evidence of osteoporosis (Figure 4.3). Many spinal osteoporotic fractures are undiagnosed at the time they occur. Consequently, thoracolumbar spine X-rays may reveal important and relatively early evidence of osteoporosis[4,5].

At an early stage, spinal radiographs may show loss of transverse trabeculae, with prominence of the vertical weight-bearing trabeculae. Later, as trabecular architecture is lost, principal X-ray appearances include wedge, crush and biconcave deformities[6]. Vertebral endplates often appear thinner and may be asymmetrically biconcave.

Radiological assessment of vertebral deformity is highly subjective and poorly reproducible. In view of the variety of fracture types, both anterior and lateral views are useful, although the majority of vertebral deformities will be visible on lateral views. The most frequently fractured vertebrae are those subject to the greatest mechanical stresses, namely T8, T12 and L1.

Because of the subjective nature of vertebral fracture reporting, considerable effort has been applied to the development of quantitative evaluation[7]. One semiquantitative system for visual grading of vertebral deformities is that according to Genant (Figure 4.4). Although such systems are not currently in widespread clinical use, their importance is likely to increase.

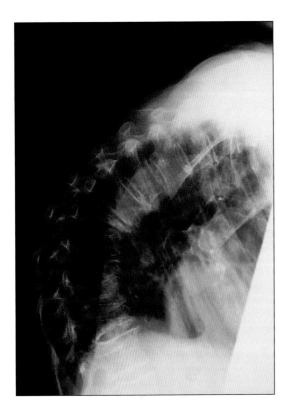

Figure 4.3 *Lateral thoracic radiograph of a patient with osteoporosis showing multiple vertebral deformities.*

Hip X-ray: Age changes in the hip demonstrate both cortical thinning and loss of trabeculae. A central area of the femoral neck (Ward's triangle) contains no trabeculae in 60% of 75-year-old women, with trabeculae being replaced by fat. X-ray appearances mirror this physiological change and the Singh index is an attempt to grade the change (Figure 4.5). This shows early loss of 'secondary' trabeculae, followed by central loss of 'tensile' trabeculae, finally followed by loss of the primary tensile group. Although of some use in population studies, such grading systems are not accurate or repeatable enough for use in the management of individual patients. Trabecular bone probably contributes to about 50% of the 'strength' of the femoral neck. and, once lost, probably cannot be replaced.

65

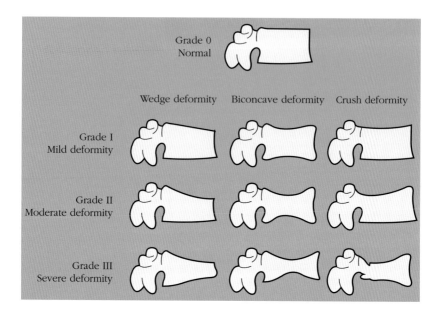

Figure 4.4 *The Genant grading system for vertebral deformity: this system assigns severity by quantifying loss of anterior, mid-, or posterior vertebral height. (Reproduced from ref. 8, with permission.)*

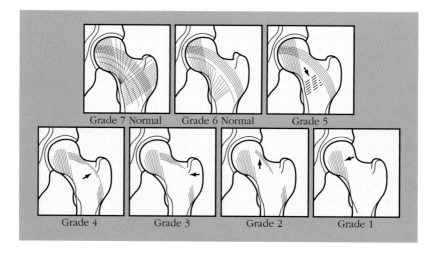

Figure 4.5 *Illustrates the trabecular grading patterns proposed by Singh et al. (Reproduced from ref. 10, with permission.)*

Bone densitometry

Imaging of the skeleton by plain radiographs has been in medical use for over 100 years. Conventional X-ray sources, however, allow only an imperfect assessment of the mineral content of a particular bone, because such sources emit X-rays of varying and unquantified energies which are variably absorbed by bone and soft tissue. The last three decades have seen major advances in our ability to quantify bone mineral non-invasively. In 1963, Cameron and Sorenson developed a method of *in vivo* measurement of bone mineral density called single photon absorptiometry (SPA)[9]. This instrument employed a sealed single energy source, but required that areas of interest be immersed in water. In 1965, dual photon absorptiometry (DPA) overcame these initial problems and enabled the measurement of bone mineral density of vertebrae (an area of interest not readily immersible). The accuracy and reproducibility of these machines was excellent but the problems associated with using a radioisotope source and diminishing source strength with time meant that widespread use of the technique was not possible. Replacement of the isotope source with an X-ray tube in 1987 overcame these problems and dual X-ray absorptiometry (DXA) became commercially viable and widely available.

X-ray absorptiometry

In X-ray absorptiometry, an X-ray tube emits photons which are collated into a single narrow beam. These pass through the skeletal site to be measured, and a monitor detects the intensity of the beam after it has passed through the body. Attenuation of the beam provides a profile of the tissues through which it has passed; attenuation is effectively zero in air and increases with passage through soft tissue.

X-ray absorptiometry may be applied to the appendicular or axial skeleton. In the appendicular skeleton, single or dual energy level X-rays may be used. The former technique is known as single energy X-ray absorptiometry (SXA). Axial sites, such as the spine and hip, are surrounded by varying amounts of soft tissue and require two levels of X-ray energy to correct for this variation (DXA). Most instruments occupy an area the size of a double bed and may therefore be used in standard sized consulting rooms (Figure 4.6). Exposure to ionising radiation is minimal (a single scan equates to about a day of normal exposure to background radiation) and the machine does not require additional protection for staff or patients. New generations of machines are available and demonstrate improved picture definition, faster scan times, and 'quick scan' facilities. Programmes are available which allow assessment of vertebral morphometry, body composition, total body bone mineral content and measurements in neonates. DXA measurements of bone mineral are highly reproducible, with precision errors (coefficient of variation) of 1–2% *in vivo*; their accuracy is somewhat lower at 5–10% (see page 74).

Hip bone density measurement: Different areas of interest within the hip may be measured (Figure 4.7).

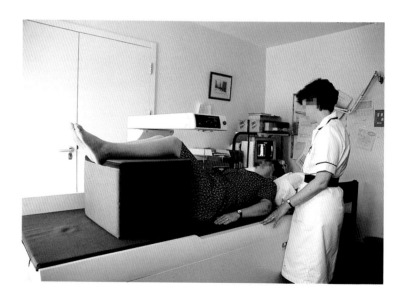

Figure 4.6 *A currently used DXA instrument. The fully-dressed subject lies above the dual X-ray source and below the mobile detector.*

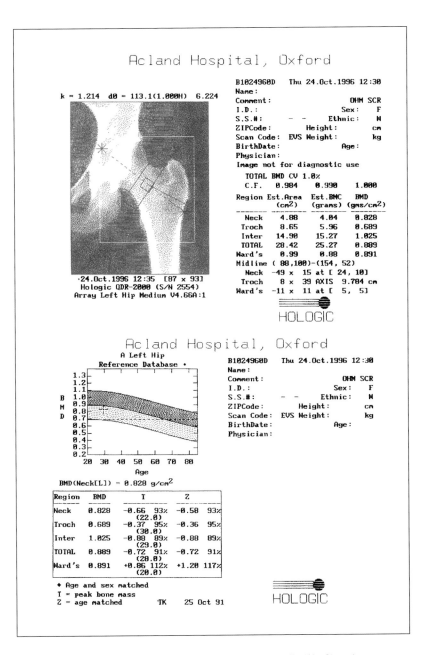

Figure 4.7 *Results of dual energy X-ray absorptiometry (DXA) of hip, showing regions of interest.*

- Femoral neck. This areas consists of more or less equal quantities of trabecular and cortical bone. A straight line is drawn through the mid-axis of the femoral neck and a 10–16 mm box is drawn perpendicular to the hip axis. The density in this area is probably the best determinant of all site fracture risk.
- Ward's triangle. This area is located in the base of the femoral neck. It has the most trabecular bone and demonstrates earliest evidence of osteoporosis, but has a high precision error.
- Intertrochanteric region (which includes part of the upper femoral shaft).
- The total value is the sum of the values of the femoral neck, trochanteric and intertrochanteric regions.

A measure of hip axis length will generally be provided. Data from the UK, USA and Australia have demonstrated that an increased hip axis length is an independent risk factor for hip fracture.

Forearm bone density measurement: The distal forearm is perhaps the quickest and easiest area of interest to measure (Figure 4.8). Small mobile densitometers exist for arm measurement only, and it may be that this approach will eventually represent a cost-effective screening tool. However, corresponding values for hip and spine are concordant in only about 70% of cases, and possibly less than this when osteoporosis exists. This means that measurement of further sites is required in most cases.

Spine bone density measurement: Vertebral fractures most frequently occur at T8, T12 and L1, where mechanical stresses are greatest (Figure 4.9). For densitometric purposes, lumbar vertebrae L1–L4 are most often measured. Where the spinal values are disproportionately high compared with vertebrae above and below, this may represent deformity, fracture or new bone formation.

Morphometric X-ray absorptiometry (MXA): With the newer generation of DXA machines it is now possible to measure vertebral dimensions and other morphometric features. Paired A/P and lateral scans covering the T4–L4 range are obtained and both views are presented simultaneously (Figure 4.10). Automatic specification of six

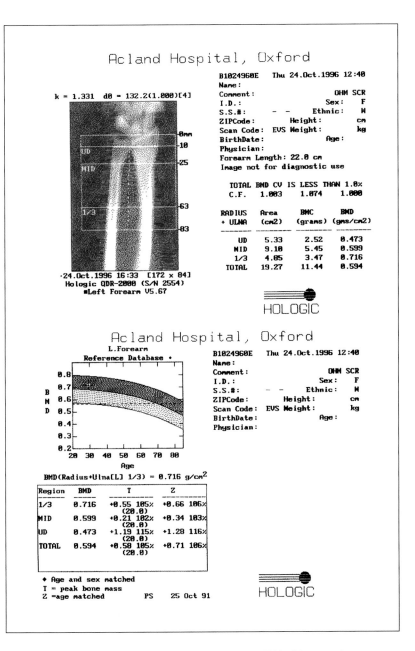

Figure 4.8 Results of single photon absorptiometry (SPA) of forearm, showing regions of interest.

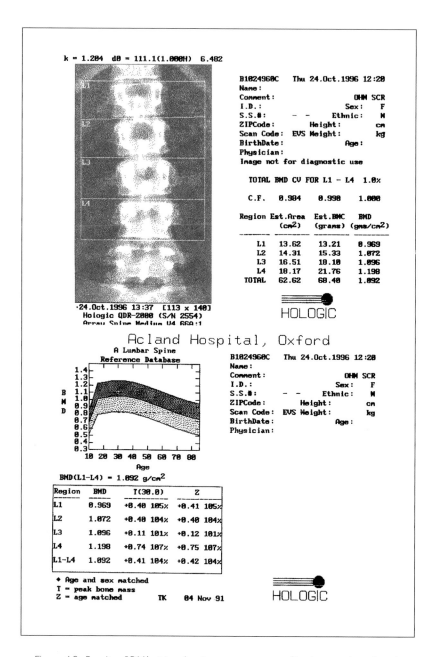

Figure 4.9 *Results of DXA spine showing measurements of lumbar vertebrae 1 to 4.*

NORTH LONDON MENOPAUSE AND OSTEOPOROSIS
STUDY CLINIC
BISHOPSWOOD HOSPITAL (01923) 834232

LATERAL SPINE MORPHOMETRY

Facility ID:

161.0cm   57.4kg   White   Female
Technician:

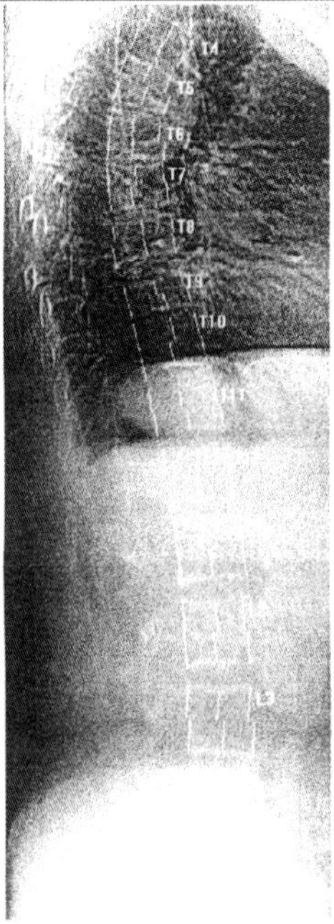

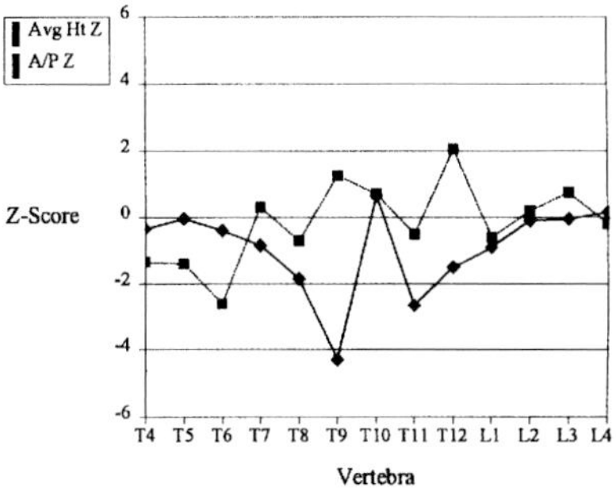

Acquired: 07/06/96 10:04:37   (1.52)
Analyzed: 07/06/96 10:10:37   (1.52)
Printed: 24/10/96 13:57:11   (1.63)
d:\archive\exp_data\jxm__400.l48

Region[1]	HEIGHT (mm)	Z	A/P Ratio	Z
T4	16.6	-0.4	0.87	-1.4
T5	17.4	-0.1	0.86	-1.4
T6	17.3	-0.4	0.77	-2.6
T7	16.9	-0.9	0.91	+0.3
T8	16.1	-1.9	0.86	-0.7
T9	13.6	-4.3	0.99	+1.3
T10	21.4	+0.7	0.98	+0.7
T11	17.8	-2.7	0.90	-0.5
T12	21.1	-1.5	1.04	+2.1
L1	23.5	-0.9	0.92	-0.6
L2	25.9	-0.1	1.00	+0.2
L3	26.5	-0.1	1.05	+0.8
L4	26.9	+0.2	1.04	-0.2

Image not for diagnosis   1-Reference based on L2, L3 and L4.
134:5.0:-10.00:70x1 -15.50:0.00 0.50x0.70 -96.00 100%
1.14:0.00   0.0:0.0   0.920:0.928   62.0:60.2

Comments: + Ve

LUNAR Expert #1148

Figure 4.10 *To demonstrate results of vertebral morphometry measurements of vertebral height.*

points on each vertebra define deformity parameters. Currently, morphometry has some advantages over X-ray in that the radiation dose is about 5% of that used for standard radiography, and that results are more reproducible. However, the lower resolution can make definition of the thoracic vertebrae difficult and sensitivity is less than for standard radiography. Radiography remains the method of choice for evaluation of spinal fracture but, as technology improves, this judgement may well reverse.

Expression of bone density measurements

From the population data shown in Figure 4.11, it is clear that BMD is distributed around a mean for a given age. An individual measurement of a given area of interest is plotted on the population graph, and an estimate of relative fracture risk is gained, as well as an assessment of the extent of bone loss. The precision (coefficient of variation) of such measures is between 0.8 and 1.5% for the spine and 1.5–3% for the hip (the term 'precision' refers to the ability of the instrument to reproduce the same results for repeated measurements of the same object). The accuracy of the measurement is between 2 and 4%. (The term accuracy refers to the ability of the instrument to produce the same result as another independent measurement method.) In this case, the ash weight may be considered to be the 'gold standard'. In most instances, serial measurements in an individual are of limited value at intervals of less than 1 year, since the annual change in bone density rarely exceeds the precision limits. The cost of an individual measurement (in 1998, in the UK) is £60–£80.

Most scans performed for clinical purposes are reported upon by an experienced physician. Such reporting is currently necessary where the experience of the referring doctor is limited. However, the need for this may decline as the technique becomes more widely available and experience increases.

Interpretation of DXA measurements: All currently available DXA machines produce computer-generated values and a constructed (computer-generated) image of the measured area. In addition, there

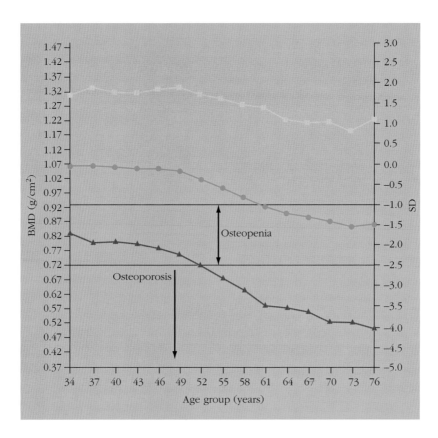

Figure 4.11 *Mean and standard deviations (SD) values, with upper and lower ranges (95% confidence limits) of bone mineral density (BMD) by age (in 3-year age bands) in 11,808 women visitors to the Bone Density Research Group, Oxford (courtesy of Dr John Shipman).*

is a population graph of BMD against age for the 'normal distribution', which the software uses as a reference range. The graph will demonstrate the mean and 1 or 2 SD deviations above and below that mean. In addition, a horizontal 'fracture risk' line will usually demarcate those values which fall more than 2 SD below the peak young adult mean (T score > –2). The values will be plotted on the graph (femoral neck, or the mean of L1–L4). The details of individual values and the image should be scrutinized, because the mean may be artificially elevated by localized abnormalities. For example, osteoarthritis with osteophyte formation may artificially elevate spinal values and mask underlying osteoporosis. Conversely, an isolated lytic lesion may, if missed, falsely suggest a diagnosis of osteoporosis.

Clinical indications for bone densitometry

Bone mineral measurements can be used for two main purposes:

■ to predict fracture risk, and

■ to measure the rate of bone loss.

The risk of fracture approximately doubles for each SD decrease in bone mineral density. Thus, a woman aged 50 years with a BMD 2 SD below average will have a 4-fold increase in lifetime risk. Bone mineral assessments at one site correlate imperfectly with measurements at other sites but, generally speaking, all techniques used for measurement of bone mass at the time of the menopause perform similarly when they are used to predict the risk of any osteoporotic fracture. However, measurements for a specific site improve the accuracy of fracture prediction at that particular site. For example, estimates of BMD at the radius or lumbar spine are associated with an approximately 1.5-fold increase in the risk of hip fracture for each SD decrease in BMD. In contrast, measurements at the hip give gradients of risk between 2.5 and 3.0. Recent data suggest a number of additional ways in which the prediction of future fracture risk using BMD measurement can be improved. These include:

■ assessment of femoral neck geometry (most notably hip axis length),

■ measurements of bone using ultrasound,

■ tests of postural stability, and

■ presence of previous fragility fractures.

In individuals with BMD above a treatment threshold in whom progressive bone loss is suspected, measurements may be repeated at intervals. The suitable interval depends upon the anticipated rate of loss and the precision error of the measurement. In general, to be significant the anticipated loss should be 2–3 times greater than the precision error, and physiological rates of loss cannot be detected in periods less than 1 year. Measurement of bone mass may also be used to monitor the treatment of osteoporosis. In such patients, including those taking hormone replacement therapy, bone mineral measurements are helpful to assess response to treatment and also to aid compliance. The effects of treatment can usually be detected within 1–2 years, depending on the agent given at the site of assessment. Treatment-induced changes are commonly most marked at the spine.

Several strategies are available for tackling the problem of osteoporosis in the population (see Chapter 5). Preventative strategies may be targeted at everyone (for example, modifications in diet, physical activity, smoking or alcohol consumption) or at high-risk subgroups. In recent years, the potential use of population-based screening using bone density measurement to target individuals at high risk has been much discussed. However, population-based screening cannot be justified at present for reasons which include the absence of a clearly-defined policy on whom to treat, what to treat with, and a validated screening programme. This should not, however, be confused with the role of BMD measurement in the diagnosis and management of osteoporosis in individual patients. The currently accepted clinical indications for bone densitometry are listed in Table 4.3.

Table 4.3 Clinical indications for bone densitometry

- Strong risk factors:
  Premature menopause
  Prolonged amenorrhoea
  Corticosteroid therapy
- Vertebral deformity/radiographic osteopenia
- Previous fragility fractures
- Monitoring of therapy

Quantitative computed tomography (QCT)

QCT can be used to determine the three dimensional image of bone at any site and to compute a true volumetric density rather than an area-based density. Standard CT instruments can be used for this purpose with the application of appropriate software. However, the high radiation exposure (50 times greater than DXA), high cost, and absence of normal ranges, have led to the technique remaining a research tool. Precision errors are higher than for DXA, at 2–4%, with accuracy quoted at between 5% and 10% when used to assess the spine. Recently, special purpose QCT scanners have been developed to measure the peripheral skeleton. The most frequently assessed site is the distal radius. Accuracy and precision are broadly similar to those for DXA.

Quantitative ultrasound assessment (QUS)

Quantitative ultrasound measurement, which remains a research tool at present, provides two indices of skeletal status:

■ BUA (broadband ultrasound attenuation), and
■ SOS (speed of sound or ultrasound velocity).

These measures are thought to give information on bone stiffness and microarchitecture in addition to bone mineral density. Ultrasound systems are portable, relatively inexpensive, involve no radiation exposure and are acceptable to the patient. Their major limitation, however, is the paucity of data assessing their accuracy and clinical utility. Two prospective studies have recently suggested that QUS may be as good as DXA in predicting hip fracture among very elderly (75+ years) subjects. However, precision error is high and it is difficult to compare results between different instruments.

Other investigative tools

Bone biopsy: Bone biopsy is rarely used in the clinical diagnosis of osteoporosis, but is helpful in detecting secondary causes of osteoporosis, such as mastocytosis, and for excluding non-osteoporotic bone disease, such as osteomalacia.

Key points

■ Increased awareness of osteoporosis is essential to detect those most at risk of fracture.

■ Dual energy X-ray absorptiometry (DXA) represents the best available measure of bone density and is the most reliable predictor of fracture risk.

■ Radiology remains the best method of diagnosing vertebral fracture.

■ Local protocols should be developed between health professionals in order to provide best care for the greatest number, and to make the best use of available resources.

References

1 Advisory Group on Osteoporosis. *Report on Osteoporosis*. Wetherby: Department of Health, 1994.

2 Kanis JA, Melton LJ, Christiansen C *et al*. The diagnosis of osteoporosis. *J Bone Mineral Research* 1993; **8**: 1137–48.

3 Delmas PD, Garnero P. Utility of biochemical markers of bone turnover. In: Marcus F, Feldman D, Kelsey J, eds. *Osteoporosis*. New York: Academic Press, 1996; 1075–88.

4 Leidig G, Storm T, Genant HK *et al*. Comparison of two methods to assess vertebral fractures. Third International Symposium on Osteoporosis, Copenhagen, Denmark, 1991; 626–8.

5 Black DM, Cummings SR, Stone K *et al*. A new approach to defining normal vertebral dimensions. *J Bone Miner Res* 1991; **6**: 883–92.

6 Smith-Bindman R, Cummings SR, Steiger P, Genant HK. A comparison of morphometric definitions of vertebral fracture. *J Bone Miner Res* 1991; **6**: 25–34.

7 Smith-Bindman R, Steiger P, Cummings SR, Genant HK. The index of radiographic area (IRA) a new approach to estimating the severity of vertebral deformity. *Bone Miner* 1991; **15**: 137–50.

8 Genant HK, Vaglar JB, Block JE. Radiology of osteoporosis. In: BL Riggs and LJ Melton, eds. *Osteoporosis, Aetiology, Diagnosis and Management*. New York: Raven Press, 1988; 181–220.

9 Cameron JR and Sorenson J. Measurement of bone mineral *in vivo*: an improved method. *Science* 1963; **143**: 230.

10 Singh M, Nagrath AR, Maini PS. Changes in trabecular pattern of the upper end of the femur as an index of osteoporosis. *J Bone Joint Surgery (Am)* 1970; **54**: 457–67.

Chapter 5

Prevention of osteoporosis

Introduction

This chapter considers various strategies for the primary prevention of osteoporosis. Secondary prevention (analogous to treatment) is considered in Chapter 6.

As a considerable amount of bone may have already been lost by the time that a fracture occurs, prevention of bone loss is likely to be a more effective strategy for reducing fracture incidence than is the treatment of established disease. There are two general strategies that may be adopted to achieve this objective — the high risk and the population approach.

In the population strategy, the object is to move the bone density distribution of the entire population in a beneficial direction. Alterations in lifestyle, such as improving nutrition, maximizing physical activity, reducing smoking and avoiding heavy alcohol consumption, fall into this category. Also important are measures to reduce the frequency of falls in the elderly, for example the removal of environmental hazards and avoidance of sedatives and hypnotics.

In the contrasting high-risk strategy, intervention is targeted at those individuals in whom fracture risk is high according to some form of screening investigation[1]. The most appropriate such screening tool, on current evidence, is bone density measurement. Although several techniques are available for this purpose, including various types of absorptiometry, computer tomography and ultrasound, the best-validated and most widely available technique is dual X-ray absorptiometry (DXA). Several prospective studies have confirmed that bone density measured by this technique is related to the risk of future fracture. The risk gradient for this relationship is similar to that between blood pressure and stroke, and there does not appear to be a threshold value for bone density above which fracture risk is stable[2]. While some studies have suggested that historical risk factors, biochemical markers of bone turnover, and ultrasound might improve fracture prediction if combined with bone densitometry, these findings are preliminary and no algorithm for their combined use in clinical practice is yet available.

The major difficulty with using the high-risk strategy to prevent osteoporotic fracture is not the screening tool, but the intervention. Most attention has been focused on the targeting of hormone replacement therapy (HRT) to women at the time of the menopause. The difficulty with this approach is that the risks and benefits of hormone replacement are predominately extraskeletal (the major potential benefit is cardiovascular protection, and the major potential hazard is breast cancer), making it inappropriate to target use simply on the basis of skeletal risk. Furthermore, bone densitometry is not sufficiently predictive of future fracture to warrant such a high-risk strategy. It is therefore widely accepted that a mass bone density screening programme to target HRT to postmenopausal women would not be an effective means of reducing fracture incidence in the general population.

Recent studies have also demonstrated that bone density measurements predict fracture risk in subjects aged 70 years and above. Novel pharmacological interventions, such as the bisphosphonates, have been shown to reduce fracture incidence in patients of this age, raising the possibility that interventions other than oestrogen might be targeted later in life, at ages when fracture incidence is rising more steeply. Studies of such strategies with the amino-bisphosphonates are already under way. Until these become available, bone density measurement is justifiable only for certain well-defined clinical indications (Chapter 4, Table 4.3), in which knowledge of the test result influences decision[3]. These clinical indications have been widely agreed, and provide the most cost-effective use of this new technology at the present time.

Identification of 'at risk' individuals

Bone loss is an asymptomatic process and in some ways can be considered clinically to be equivalent to hypertension. In each case, patients present to the health care system when a complication arises, either fracture in the case of osteoporosis, or stroke in hypertension. The key in each case is early identification of the patients at greatest risk, identifying those for intervention.

As in many other disorders of ageing, a large number of risk factors have been incriminated in the pathogenesis of osteoporosis among the elderly (Table 5.1). Some clearly change the onset, duration or rate of bone loss in individuals, whereas others increase fracture risk by modifying the risk of injury. Yet others may be linked by an association that is statistically significant without any cause–effect relationship. Only relatively few are of value clinically, and even these suffer from the difficulties inherent in translating epidemiological data into clinical practice. The most frequently cited risk factors fall into four broad groups:

- genetic
- nutritional
- lifestyle
- endocrine.

Superimposed on these are a variety of sporadic factors that can affect the skeleton, including chronic illness, disuse, and a wide variety of drugs (most notably corticosteroids).

In general, for each patient, the more risk factors present and the longer the duration of their presence, the greater the risk of future problems. Physicians can use the presence of these factors in two ways:

- they can be used to alert the patient and physician to the likelihood of osteoporosis, and
- those risk factors that are amenable to elimination or alteration should be discussed with the patient.

Table 5.1 Factors contributing to osteoporosis

Genetic
- White or Asian ethnicity
- Family (maternal) history of fractures
- Small body frame
- Long hip axis

Lifestyle and nutritional
- Premature menopause (< 45 years)
- Nulliparity
- Late menarche
- Prolonged secondary amenorrhoea
- Smoking
- Excessive alcohol intake
- Inactivity
- Prolonged immobilization
- Prolonged parenteral nutrition
- Low body weight

Medical disorders
- Anorexia nervosa
- Malabsorption due to gastrointestinal and hepatobiliary diseases
- Primary hyperparathyroidism
- Thyrotoxicosis
- Primary hypogonadism
- Prolactinoma
- Hypercortisolism
- Osteogenesis imperfecta
- Rheumatoid arthritis
- Chronic obstructive lung disease
- Chronic neurological disorders
- Chronic renal failure

Table 5.1 (Contd.)

- Mastocytosis
- Type 1 diabetes
- Organ transplantation

Drugs
- Chronic corticosteroid therapy
- Excessive thyroid therapy
- Anticoagulants
- Chemotherapy
- Gonadotrophin-releasing hormone agonist or antagonist
- Anticonvulsants

Practically, the menopause in women is the usual time when evaluation of the patient for osteoporosis begins, although nutritional and lifestyle habits should be changed as early in life as possible.

No combination of these risk factors is a surrogate for bone densitometry, but risk factor review is a useful initial approach to any patient. The analogy is, again, hypertension for which there is also a list of risk factors, but no assemblage of these predicts an individual patient's blood pressure well enough to warrant treatment.

Finally, a number of factors which relate to trauma will influence the risk of sustaining an osteoporotic fracture. These include the risk of falls, their severity and the neuromuscular response to them.

Measures to diminish osteoporosis

Exercise

Exercise is important in the prevention of osteoporotic fractures through its influence on both bone density and the risk of falls. Weight-bearing physical activity is associated with increased peak bone density[4]. There

85

are several studies relating physical activity in elderly subjects to bone density at various skeletal sites. Although the results of these studies are inconsistent, greater physical activity tends to be associated with greater bone density. In addition, some (but not all) controlled trials of exercise regimens have demonstrated improvements in bone density. The most successful regimens appear to be those in which high-amplitude loading cycles are applied discontinuously to bone. However, epidemiological studies uniformly suggest a reduction in the risk of hip fracture from regular weight-bearing physical activity[5]. This intervention is beneficial from cardiovascular and psychological standpoints also, and constitutes a prudent public health measure in the general population.

Changing the pattern of physical activity may be difficult, especially for patients who are not positively motivated. This is especially true when discussing prevention with patients who are, by definition, asymptomatic. Many outpatients have relatively low levels of fitness and require formal cardiovascular evaluation before beginning an exercise programme. It is suggested that, to improve compliance, the exercise activity chosen should be fun. Generally, any weight bearing will be of benefit to the skeleton. Recreational therapy, which has a social component, may serve to improve patient compliance. However, even simple activities, such as walking, are useful and can be added to the daily routine with minimal difficulty. Back-strengthening exercises are probably also of value and patients may be referred to a physiotherapist for specific instructions.

Calcium intake

Adequate calcium nutrition is important in promoting peak bone density and in preventing bone loss. The dietary requirements for calcium increase at puberty, when some studies have demonstrated that a total intake of up to 1200 mg daily may be required for maximal skeletal benefit. Randomized controlled trials (RCTs) also suggest that calcium supplementation reduces bone loss when compared with a placebo[5,6]. This intervention appears most beneficial to subjects with a low calcium intake, and to women who are more than 5 years postmenopausal. Finally, a prospective RCT among institutionalized elderly people in France suggested that a combination of calcium and vitamin D supplementation reduced hip fracture risk over a 3-year period[7]. This observation is in accord with the hypothesis that hypovitaminosis D is an important risk fracture for hip fracture in the elderly, through its association with osteomalacia, secondary hyperparathyroidism, and proximal myopathy. However, the use of vitamin D supplementation alone among the institutionalized elderly did not reduce hip fracture risk in a Dutch RCT[8]. Until the appropriate dosing regimen and formulation for the correction of hypovitaminosis D in this population is established, it would seem sensible to aim at a dietary calcium intake of 800 mg daily for British adults, with physiological doses of vitamin D for all elderly people.

There is controversy over population recommendations on dietary calcium intake. In providing advice, the intent is to ensure that the majority of the population obtain sufficient calcium to maintain calcium balance. US recommendations include an intake of 800 mg until age 10 years, 1500 mg during adolescence and 1200 mg thereafter, increasing to 1500 mg during pregnancy and lactation, and if at increased risk of osteoporosis. To achieve such intakes, it is commonly necessary to resort to calcium supplementation and most individuals require only 500–1000 mg daily as a supplement to dietary sources to achieve these intakes. There are many forms of calcium available as supplements, and advice to the patient should be as simple as possible. First, it is important that the calcium is bioavailable. Studies suggest that proprietary forms are, in general, more available than non-proprietary varieties; although some of the latter are clearly adequate, in general the former are preferred. Because calcium absorption is better in an acid environment for the carbonate, it is usually recommended that the supplement is taken with food. The addition of a modest calcium supplement to each meal is a regimen to which the patient can easily adhere. The elemental content of calcium varies with the product: calcium carbonate contains 40% elemental calcium by weight, calcium phosphate 31%, calcium lactate 13% and calcium gluconate 9%. Absorption of the calcium as citrate is slightly more efficient and not dependent on acidity. Importantly, the cost of calcium supplements should be considered.

At the recommended dietary intakes, calcium supplementation is virtually free of side effects. If eructation, intestinal colic and constipation occur with the carbonate, citrate is a useful alternative.

Lifestyle modification

Heavy alcohol consumption and cigarette smoking are both known to influence bone loss, and should be actively discouraged to prevent osteoporosis. In addition, risk factors for falls should be corrected among elderly people. These include the elimination of environmental hazards such as loose rugs and poor lighting, as well as the correction of age-related disorders such as deficits in vision and hearing.

Using HRT in appropriate patients

HRT prevents further loss of bone mineral at all skeletal sites, and many case–control and cohort studies suggest that post menopausal use of oestrogen is associated with a reduction in fracture risk[9]. However, the duration of treatment required for anti-fracture efficacy remains uncertain. The lower limit of this duration is known to be around 10 years, but there is increasing evidence that bone loss recommences at a rapid rate when therapy is stopped and life-long treatment might be necessary for continued benefit.

The decision to utilize HRT depends upon a number of factors including the following:

- evidence of hypogonadal status
- the absence of absolute contraindications to treatment
- the risks and benefits of HRT for the individual
- the acceptability of long-term HRT to the patient.

The assessment of gonadal status is not usually difficult. The presence of postmenopausal symptoms is presumptive evidence of oestrogen deficiency in hysterectomized women. In some women, biochemical evaluation of gonadal function by the measurement of gonadotrophins (luteinizing hormone and follicle-stimulating hormone) is required. There are few absolute contraindications to oestrogen therapy (Table 5.2).

Table 5.2 Potential, relative and absolute contraindications for hormone replacement therapy

Absolute contraindications
- Active endometrial or breast cancer
- Pregnancy
- Undiagnosed abnormal vaginal bleeding
- Severe active liver disease
- Acute deep venous thrombosis and thromboembolic disease
- Recent hormone-dependent cancers

Relative contraindications (specialist opinion may be sought)
- Uncontrolled hypertension
- Previous spontaneous deep venous thrombosis or pulmonary embolism
- Systemic lupus erythematosis
- Endometriosis
- Fibroids
- Previous breast cancer or strong family history of breast cancer
- Endometrial cancer (within 5 years)

Potential contraindications*
- Migraine
- Diabetes
- Pre-existing gall stones
- Mild liver disease

*Transdermal route preferred.

These include active endometrial or breast cancer, undiagnosed abnormal vaginal bleeding and thromboembolic disease. There are, in addition, several situations where a careful assessment is appropriate and in some instances might require referral to a specialist.

These include:

■ uncontrolled hypertension

■ previous history of pulmonary embolism

■ systemic lupus erythematosus

■ endometriosis

■ fibroids

■ previous breast cancer or a strong family history of the disorder.

The risks and benefits of HRT should be explained to patients. The major benefits of long-term oestrogen use are a reduction in the risk of cardiovascular disease and of osteoporotic fracture (Figures 5.1, 5.2). The major adverse consequence is a small increase in the risk of breast cancer (Figure 5.3). The increase in breast cancer risk is lower than the risk of breast cancer associated with obesity, regular alcohol intake or a family history. In addition, the reported increase in some studies has not been associated with an increase in mortality and might stem from the improved gynaecological surveillance that occurs among women using HRT.

Analyses indicate that the benefits of HRT outweigh the risks when mortality is used as the indicator of outcome. However, after explanation of the risks and benefits many women prefer to avoid HRT and alternative options should be discussed. Recent studies also suggest a small increase in the risk of thromboembolism and a protective effect against Alzheimer's disease (see Chapter 6).

So-called natural oestrogens (those found in living organisms) such as 17β-oestradiol, are preferable to synthetic oestrogens such as mestranol and ethinyloestradiol. The bone-sparing dose of oestradiol is 2 mg daily, while that of conjugated equine oestrogen is 0.625 mg daily (Tables 5.3, 5.4). Hysterectomized women can be given oestrogen preparations alone. Women with a uterus should be given a combined oestrogen and progestogen, which prevents the occurrence of endometrial hyperplasia and reduces the risk of endometrial carcinoma.

The side effects of HRT include menstrual or breakthrough bleeding in non-hysterectomized women, breast tenderness, a bloated feeling and increase in weight.

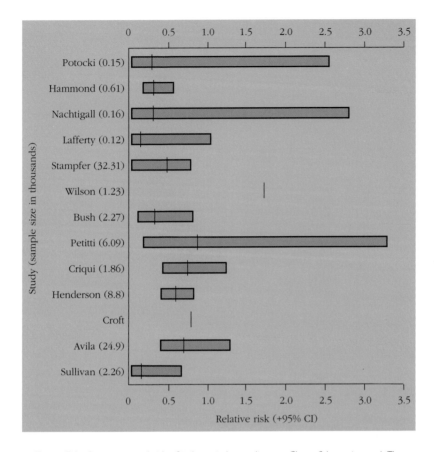

Figure 5.1 *Oestrogen and risk of ischaemic heart disease. CI, confidence interval. The figure shows that the relative risk of cardiovascular disease is below 1.0 in almost all the studies, with an average value of around 0.75. (Reproduced from Smith R, Studd J. The Menopause and HRT. London: Martin Dunitz, 1993, with permission.)*

Oestrogens and progestogens are usually given by mouth (Table 5.5). Transdermal and cutaneous delivery systems bypass the liver; these routes may be advantageous in patients with -mild liver disease or gall stones. There is no evidence that transdermal oestrogen has greater efficacy than orally administered preparations.

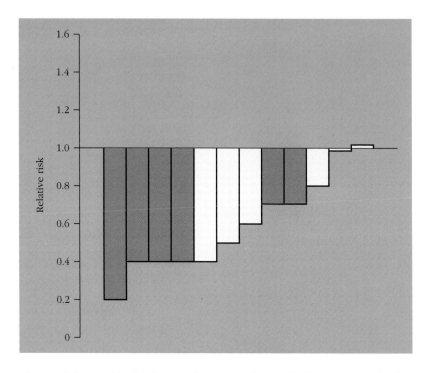

Figure 5.2 *Relative risk of hip fracture after oestrogen therapy. The figure shows the diversity of results in case control and cohort studies, with greater protection generally observed in the latter. Relative risk (RR) of 1.0 implies no difference in fracture risk compared with a control group.* ■ *Case control study;* □ *cohort study. (Reproduced from ref. 9, with permission.)*

Continuous combined oestrogen and progestogen regimens are also available (Table 5.6). These are particularly suitable for postmenopausal, rather than perimenopausal, women in whom withdrawal bleeds are not tolerated. These regimens generally do not induce cyclical bleeding and suppress endometrial proliferation. However, in about one-quarter of women irregular bleeding may occur, particularly soon after the onset of treatment. This can be minimized by increasing the dose of progestogen, where oestrogen and progestogen are being used separately.

Topical oestrogen vaginal creams, pessaries and tablets have a potent local action and effectively relieve vaginal dryness and atrophic vaginitis. The rate of absorption of oestrogens from the vagina varies considerably, depending on the state of the tissue and the formulation

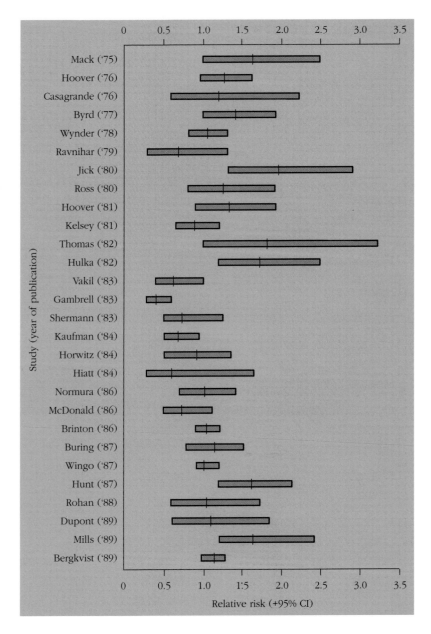

Figure 5.3 *HRT and incidence of breast cancer. The figure shows wide variation in relative risk, based on 5–10 years of oestrogen use. A recent analysis suggests a risk increase of 2.3% for each year on therapy, although mortality from breast cancer appears unaffected. (Reproduced from Smith R, Studd J.* The Menopause and HRT. *London: Martin Dunitz, 1993, with permission.)*

93

Table 5.3 Bone-sparing doses of commonly used preparations

Oestrogen preparations	Bone-sparing dose (mg per day)
Oestradiol	2
Oestradiol valerate	2
Piperazine oestrone sulphate	1.5
Conjugated equine oestrogens	0.625
Oestradiol implants (6-monthly)	50
Oestradiol cream	1.5–3
Transdermal oestradiol	0.05
Ethinyl oestradiol	0.025
Oestrone sulphate	1.25
Other agents	
Tibolone	2.5
Progestogen preparations (given for 12–14 days out of 28 days with continuous oestrogen)	
Norethisterone (Norethindrone)	0.7
Di-norgestrel	0.075–0.15
Medroxyprogesterone acetate*	5–10
Dydrogesterone	10
Megestrol	80

*Commonly used in the USA.

used. Where significant absorption occurs, cyclical progestogens may be needed, particularly with dienoestrol or Premarin cream. Oestrogel is a newly developed oestrogen gel which may be particularly useful for those who cannot use oral formulations or patches.

Table 5.4 Different oestrogens used in HRT

Low dose	Intermediate dose	High dose
Conjugated equine oestrogens 0.625 mg	Estraderm TTS 100 μg	Oestradiol implant 75 mg decreasing to 50 mg long-term maintenance dose
Conjugated equine oestrogens 1.25 mg	Oestradiol implant 50 mg decreasing to 25 mg long-term maintenance dose	
Oestradiol valerate 1 mg		
Oestradiol valerate 2 mg		
Estraderm TTS 50 μg		
Evorel 50 μg		

Tibolone is a synthetic analogue of the gonadal steroids with combined oestrogenic, progestogenic and androgenic properties (Table 5.6). The parent compound appears to bind preferentially with oestrogen receptors, whereas its metabolites have greater affinity for progesterone and androgen receptors. It prevents experimentally induced oestrogen-deficiency osteoporosis and does not cause endometrial hyperplasia in the doses used in women. It is effective in controlling hot flushes, sweats and mood, and recent studies suggest that it prevents postmenopausal bone loss. It should be used only in women who are at least 1 year postmenopausal. In those women who change from combined HRT to tibolone, cyclical progestogens should be given until the withdrawal bleed ceases. The long-term effects on cardiovascular morbidity have not been evaluated, but tibolone decreases both high-density lipoprotein and VLDL and may increase insulin resistance.

Table 5.5 Modes of administration of HRT

Type of HRT	Advantages	Disadvantages
Oral	Familiar	Poor compliance
	Flexible	First-pass hepatic effect
	Inexpensive	
Non-oral		
■ Oestrogen patches	No first-pass hepatic effect	Skin reactions
		Adhesion problems
■ Oestrogen implants	Compliance	Minor surgical procedure
	No first-pass hepatic effect	
	Testosterone replacement can be given by implant also	

Table 5.6 Examples of 'no bleed' therapies

Brand name	Manufacturer	Active ingredient and dose
Livial	Organon, Cambridge	Tibolone 2.5 mg daily
Kliofem	Novo Nordisk, Crawley, West Sussex	Oestradiol 2 mg/ norethisterone 1 mg daily
Premique	Wyeth, Maidenhead, Berkshire	Conjugated equine oestrogens 0.625 mg/MPA* 5 mg daily

*MPA, medroxyprogesterone acetate.

Other drug therapy

The last decade of the twentieth century has witnessed the emergence of several pharmacological agents that retard bone loss. These include the following:

- the bisphosphonates
- calcitonin
- calcitriol
- low-dose sodium fluoride.

Other agents, most notably the selective oestrogen receptor modulators (SERMS), are in advanced stages of clinical evaluation. Recent data suggest that raloxifene, one of the selective oestrogen receptor modulators, retards bone loss in postmenopausal women, exerts a beneficial effect on lipid profile, and might even reduce the risk of breast cancer.

All of these agents are likely to be more useful in the treatment of established osteoporosis, where fractures have already occurred. Their role in the primary prevention of bone loss (with the possible exception of the SERMS) is much less certain. Studies have demonstrated that calcium, the bisphosphonates (cyclical etidronate therapy and alendronate) and calcitonin are effective in retarding bone loss among postmenopausal women. However, few of these studies have been large or protracted enough to demonstrate anti-fracture efficacy convincingly when used in the sixth decade of life. RCTs using these agents for the treatment of established disease have tended to confirm anti-fracture efficacy. It therefore seems reasonable to consider these alternatives to oestrogen among postmenopausal women who wish to protect themselves against osteoporosis, but cannot (or do not wish to) take HRT. These agents will also have clinical uses for the prevention of bone loss among men who are at increased risk of osteoporosis.

Key points

■ Osteoporosis is an important clinical problem through its association with age-related fractures.

■ The prevention of osteoporosis can be viewed at the level of the population and the individual.

■ Mass screening using bone densitometry to target hormone replacement therapy (HRT) is not justifiable; the technology is most effectively used for certain specific clinical indications in which decisions rest upon the result.

■ Public health measures to maintain physical activity, maximize dietary calcium intake, avoid tobacco and excessive alcohol use, and prevent the risk of falls in the elderly, should be encouraged in order to reduce the risk of fractures in the population as a whole.

■ HRT is an effective means of retarding bone loss among postmenopausal women. However, the risks and benefits of HRT are complex and should be discussed on an individual basis.

■ Several other agents are now available that prevent further fractures in individuals with established osteoporosis. These alternatives to HRT will be increasingly used in the primary prevention of osteoporosis.

References

1 Cooper C, Melton LJ. Epidemiology of osteoporosis. *Trends Endocrinol Metab* 1992; **3**: 224–9.

2 Cooper C, Aihie A. Osteoporosis: recent advances in pathogenesis and treatment. *Q J Med* 1994; **87**: 203–9.

3 Compston JE, Cooper C, Kanis J. Bone densitometry in clinical practice. *Br Med J* 1995; **310**: 1507–10.

4 Cooper C, Eastell R. Bone gain and loss in premenopausal women. *Br Med J* 1993; **306**: 1357–8.

5 Cooper C. Osteoporosis. In: Hochberg M, Silman A J, eds. *Epidemiology of the Rheumatic Diseases*. Oxford: Oxford University Press, 1993; 422–64.

6 Compston JE. The role of vitamin D and calcium supplementation in the prevention of osteoporotic fractures in the elderly. *Clin Endocrinol* 1995; **43**: 393–405.

7 Chapuy MC, Arlot M, Duboeuf F *et al.* Vitamin D3 and calcium to prevent hip fracture in the elderly. *N Engl J Med* 1992; **327**: 1537–42.

8 Lips P, Graafmans W, Ooms M, Bezemer D, Bouter L. Vitamin D supplementation and fracture incidence in elderly persons. *Ann Intern Med* 1996; **124**: 400–6.

9 Gallagher JC. Oestrogen: prevention and treatment of osteoporosis. In: Marcus R, Feldman D, Kelsey J, eds. *Osteoporosis*. New York: Academic Press, 1996; 1191–208.

Chapter 6

Treatment of osteoporosis

Introduction

Prevention and treatment of osteoporosis are conventionally dealt with separately. This is largely an artificial distinction, since loss of bone is continuous and the methods used in the prevention of this loss and its subsequent treatment overlap[1-4]. These issues are fully discussed by Marcus *et al.*[5] in their recent textbook on osteoporosis.

The amount of bone in the skeleton at any age in maturity depends on the amount of bone present in early adulthood (peak bone mass) and its subsequent loss (Chapter 2). The present chapter is primarily concerned with the prevention of further bone loss and attempts at its restoration. It will be recalled that the amount of bone depends on the balance between new bone formation by osteoblasts and the breakdown of bone by osteoclasts. In theory, therefore, bone mass can still be conserved by increasing formation rate or decreasing the rate of resorption, or both (Table 6.1).

In practice there are very few ways of increasing bone formation, apart from mechanical stress (see below) and the administration of fluoride; therefore, the current drug treatment of osteoporosis centres around the reduction of resorption. The effectiveness of this is strictly limited and depends on the architectural state of bone, its rate of turnover and the agent used (Figure 6.1).

In osteoporosis, bone is lost in two main ways[6]. This is well demonstrated by scanning electron microscopic examination of trabecular bone (Figure 6.2). The trabeculae not only become thinner

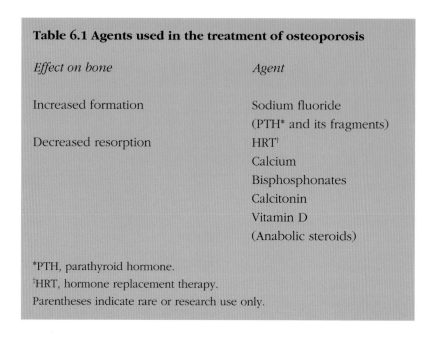

Table 6.1 Agents used in the treatment of osteoporosis

Effect on bone	*Agent*
Increased formation	Sodium fluoride
	(PTH* and its fragments)
Decreased resorption	HRT†
	Calcium
	Bisphosphonates
	Calcitonin
	Vitamin D
	(Anabolic steroids)

*PTH, parathyroid hormone.
†HRT, hormone replacement therapy.
Parentheses indicate rare or research use only.

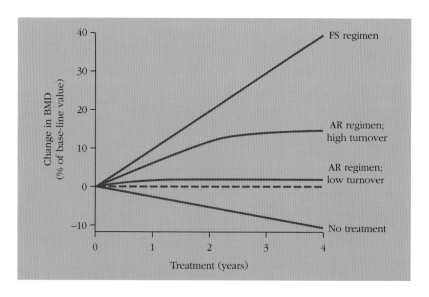

Figure 6.1 *Theoretical patterns of change in bone mineral density (BMD) with formation-stimulating (FS) and antiresponsive (AR) regimens (see text). (Reproduced from ref. 1, with permission.)*

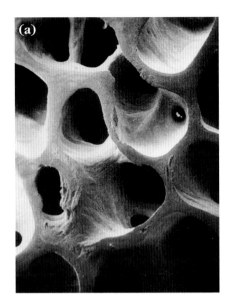
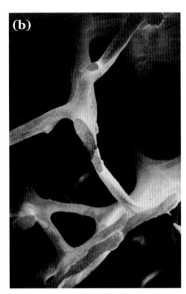

Figure 6.2 *Scanning electron microscopic appearances of (a) normal and (b) osteoporotic trabecular bone. The bone in (b) from a postmenopausal woman shows thinning of the trabeculae with loss of connectivity and plate perforation. (Reproduced from ref. 2, with permission.)*

but they may also be perforated by aggressive resorption (Figure 6.3). Although it is, in theory, possible to increase the thickness of trabeculae, it is unlikely that the continuity of broken trabeculae can be restored[6].

The usual effect of an antiresorptive agent is to produce a temporary increase in measured bone mineral density (BMD) in the first 1–2 years, after which a plateau or resumed loss occurs (Figures 6.1, 6.4). One explanation for this is that initially the bone antiresorptive agent dissociates the activities of the osteoclast and osteoblast in such a way that resorption ceases and the remaining cavities are filled in with bone produced by osteoblasts[2]. Subsequently, new bone formation falls as the osteoblasts detect (probably by biochemical messages) the reduced activity of the osteoclasts, no further resorption cavities remain to be refilled, and

103

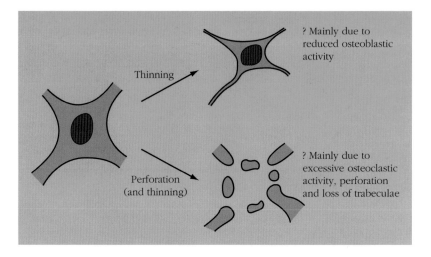

Figure 6.3 *Diagram to show how trabecular bone may be lost in osteoporosis. (Adapted from ref. 6.)*

bone turnover rate falls. The reason for this apparent waning of the effect of an antiresorptive agent is not fully understood. The effect of an antiresorptive agent will also depend on the initial rate of bone turnover (being more effective where bone turnover is increased), the number of resorbing sites and the agent used (Figure 6.1). The magnitude and duration of the initial increase in bone density seem too great to be explained entirely by the refilling of the increased numbers of resorption cavities present when the bone turnover rate is high. Long-term studies of antiresorptive agents are not always available and most deal with bone density but not fracture rate. Some antiresorptive agents may also have anabolic as well as antiresorptive effects.

Stimulation of bone formation
Exercise
Mechanical stress on the skeleton increases the activity of the osteoblasts and increases bone mass or slows its loss at any age[7]. The effect is more marked in the young skeleton and virtually

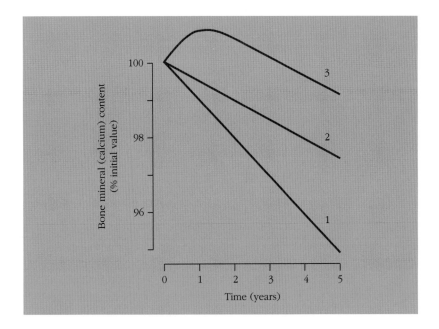

Figure 6.4 *Relationship between bone mineral content and rate of bone turnover. Line 1 shows a 1% annual loss; reduction of bone turnover by 50% halves the rate of bone loss (line 2); line 3 shows the temporary effect of an antiresorptive agent. (Reproduced from Kanis JA, Aaron J, Thavarajah M et al. Osteoporosis: causes and therapeutic implications. In: Smith R, ed. Osteoporosis 1990. Royal College of Physicians Publications, 1990; 45–56, with permission).*

undetectable in the old. Even where the exercise-produced changes in bone density are very small, there are important cardiovascular advantages that should not be disregarded. The way in which mechanical signals stimulate the osteoblasts is unknown. There is evidence that the osteocytes (within mineralized bone) are important in this regard and act as a sensing system to convert mechanical stimuli into mitogenic messengers (see Chapter 2).

The mechanical signals that are most effective are weight-bearing and varied. This is confirmed by measurement of BMD at the stressed site. The long-term effects of exercise on the human skeleton and on fracture rate are not known; likewise, it is not known what happens to bone density when an exercise regimen is stopped.

Fluoride

It has been known for many years that oral sodium fluoride can produce a progressive and sustained increase in bone mass and hence in measured vertebral BMD. At cellular level it selectively stimulates the activity of the osteoblasts which, however, produce a woven type of bone that is structurally unsound. This change may differ from one part of the skeleton to another. Thus, there is no decrease in spinal fracture rate and possibly an increase in peripheral fractures in subjects on fluoride. Side effects include gastrointestinal problems and lower extremity pain syndrome. These conclusions have been drawn from some studies in America (fluoride dose 75 mg/day). Experience from France (where a smaller dose is used) is more encouraging. Likewise, a slow-release preparation of 25 mg twice daily increased spinal and femoral neck bone mass and reduced the frequency of new vertebral fractures. Currently, sodium fluoride is not used in the UK to treat osteoporosis but it has received a licence in the United States[8,9,10].

Other agents

Parathyroid hormone in low doses can increase BMD, because of its anabolic effect on bone, but this has been demonstrated only in a research setting[11]. As with fluoride, there is some evidence of a redistribution of bone throughout the skeleton. Growth factors such as insulin-like growth factors, bone morphogenetic proteins and transforming growth factor-β could be useful in the future, provided that they could be easily administered and targeted to the skeleton so that any increase in bone and mineralization would be restricted to the normal skeleton, and provided that they were free from side effects (Chapter 7).

Antiresorptive agents

Hormone replacement therapy (see also Chapter 5)

The effectiveness of oestrogen replacement in preventing bone loss in postmenopausal women is now well established[3], together with epidemiological evidence of reduced rates of hip fracture[5]. Initial studies were carried out on young women who had had both a hysterectomy and bilateral oophorectomy and who, in the absence of oestrogen, lost bone rapidly.

Since oestrogen replacement increases the incidence of endometrial cancer and this effect can be abolished by giving progestogen, women who have not had a hysterectomy require both oestrogen and progestogen (Chapter 5).

The effects and advantages of hormone replacement therapy (HRT) have been demonstrated most convincingly in hysterectomized women on oestrogen alone[12]. In this group not only does oestrogen prevent bone loss but it also produces significant long-term cardiovascular advantages. It may also have a beneficial effect on Alzheimer's disease[13]. It is not clear whether progestogen (given to those with an intact uterus) abolishes or modifies these advantages, but preliminary evidence suggests that this is unlikely.

A complication of HRT that is difficult to assess is the possibility of breast cancer. During the first 10 years of treatment, mortality from breast cancer is probably not increased; after this time the mean relative risk may be 1.5, with very wide 95% confidence limits[14] (Figure 5.3). Likewise there is very recent evidence of a slight increase in thromboembolism in postmenopausal women given HRT[15].

For hysterectomized women the skeletal and cardiovascular advantages of HRT outweigh the possible disadvantages of increased breast cancer; for women with an intact uterus the balance is altered, and HRT is also less acceptable since it is usually associated with cyclical bleeding. Since HRT is usually not given for more than 10 years, and since bone appears to be lost rapidly when HRT is stopped, so that by the age of 70 the bone density does not differ between those who have had HRT and those who have not, there is clearly a difficulty in deciding on the optimum age to give hormone replacement (see p.116).

A distinction is made between giving HRT early in the menopause to prevent bone loss and fracture (Chapter 5) and giving HRT in established osteoporosis to prevent further bone loss (and marginally to increase BMD) and to reduce future fracture rate. There is now good evidence that HRT has both of these effects.

Calcium

For decades there has been a controversy about the relation of calcium deficiency to osteoporosis and the possibility of preventing bone loss by giving extra calcium[16]. In the background to this controversy, it is known that in postmenopausal women with oestrogen deficiency there is defective calcium absorption and negative calcium balance. Since there is also bone loss at the same time, it was reasonable to consider that the osteoporosis is due to the malabsorption of calcium and that increasing calcium intake should therefore reduce the rate of bone loss. Another possibility exists, however — namely, that the negative calcium balance is the result of the bone loss, in which case giving calcium would not be expected to have an effect on bone loss. Measurement of bone density by DXA has made it possible to show that additional calcium may increase peak bone mass and slow bone loss[4,17]; further, together with vitamin D in physiological amounts, it appears to reduce fracture rate[18]. Thus, studies on identical twins have shown that the rate of increase of BMD is greater in twins given additional calcium[19], and similar results have been obtained in adolescent non-twin girls[20]. However, it is not clear how long this benefit is maintained.

In women after the menopause, the daily addition of 1000 mg (or more) of oral calcium can slow axial or appendicular bone loss under certain circumstances[17]. Further, calcium supplements given to late menopausal women on a low (less than 400 mg daily) calcium intake reduce the rate of bone loss. The effect of oral calcium on bone loss is not dramatic and is more effective when combined with other measures aimed to preserve the skeleton, such as exercise or vitamin D. Thus, when additional calcium is combined with exercise it can prevent bone loss in postmenopausal women[21]. The recent work on the skeletal effects of calcium has been reviewed, and none of the results should be accepted uncritically[17,22].

Bisphosphonates

Bisphosphonates are based on a P-C-P chemical background and are analogues of pyrophosphate that are not destroyed by naturally

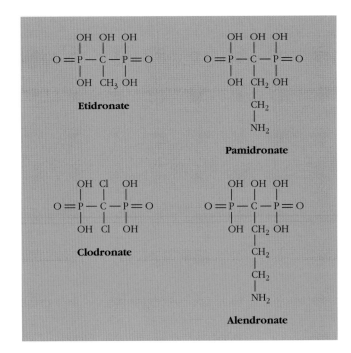

Figure 6.5
*Basic
structure of
bisphos-
phonates.*

occurring pyrophosphatases (Figure 6.5). Their mode of action is not known in detail but their main effect is to reduce osteoclast-mediated bone resorption. The first bisphosphonate used clinically (in Paget's disease) was disodium etidronate (EHDP; Didronel) and until recently was the only bisphosphonate licensed for use in osteoporosis. In Paget's disease the large doses given initially produced a mineralization defect similar to osteomalacia. In osteoporosis a far smaller dose is given cyclically with calcium and there is little or no consistent evidence of defective mineralization. Other bisphosphonates include pamidronate, ibandronate, tiludronate, risedronate and alendronate. Alendronate, like pamidronate, is an amino-bisphosphonate.

Initial studies on the skeletal effects of cyclical etidronate showed an increase in vertebral BMD and a decrease in vertebral fracture rate without any significant effect on the rest of the skeleton. The increase in BMD in the first 2 years of treatment is compatible with the known

109

effect of an antiresorptive agent on the bone remodelling cycle. The question currently under investigation is whether this increase will be maintained in subsequent years, with beneficial effects on the skeleton and sustained reduction in fracture rate[23]; recent results suggest that this is, in fact, the case[24].

Considerable interest is now focused on alendronate (under the name of Fosamax). This potent aminobisphosphonate has a selective effect on bone resorption with no deleterious effect on mineralization. It is effective orally but, like all bisphosphonates, is poorly absorbed. It reduces bone resorption and increases BMD; results from large trials show a significant reduction in vertebral and hip fracture rate although the number of peripheral fractures remains small[25,26].

Calcitonin

The main effect of administered calcitonin is to suppress osteoclastic activity. As a result, it temporarily increases BMD. Unfortunately, until recently it needed to be given by injection and had significant side effects including nausea, shivering and 'flu-like symptoms. Other preparations are now available, including a nasal spray and suppositories. Their effect on the skeleton has yet to be established convincingly. However, calcitonin is widely used in continental European countries, in a dose of 50 IU daily or every other day. Injected calcitonin also appears to have an analgesic effect and is sometimes used to treat the pain of vertebral fracture.

Vitamin D

Elderly people, particularly those constantly living indoors, tend to become vitamin D deficient, as shown by a low concentration of 25-hydroxycholecalciferol (25-(OH)D) in the plasma, and a small proportion may develop osteomalacia. It has been suggested that, in such people, parathyroid-mediated bone resorption stimulated by hypocalcaemia may also lead to osteoporosis and that this may be prevented by increasing intestinal absorption of calcium by giving vitamin D. There is evidence that giving vitamin D can reduce the observed winter-time bone loss in those living in the northern hemisphere[27], and that giving both calcium and vitamin D to elderly women may reduce the risk of hip and non-vertebral fracture[18]. The amount of vitamin D given should be in the physiological range (up to 1000 IU = 25 μg daily).

The use of vitamin D metabolites calcitriol and alphacalcidol has been extensively reviewed by Reid[28]. Where there is clear evidence of vitamin D deficiency, physiological doses of native vitamin D are appropriate and where there is reason to consider that 1 α-hydroxylation of 25-(OH)D is defective, as in renal failure, then a 1 α-hydroxylated metabolite (calcitriol or alphacalcidol) is appropriate. As 1 α-hydroxylation may become less efficient with age, a case could be made to give calcitriol or alphacalcidol to reduce postmenopausal bone loss. However, the evidence that this is more effective than native vitamin D is slight.

Other possible useful agents
Clearly, when there is sex hormone deficiency other than that at the menopause, oestrogen replacement is also appropriate; similarly, in men with testosterone deficiency this hormone should be replaced. The role of androgens and anabolic agents in postmenopausal osteoporosis is not established[29]. Anabolic steroids are related to androgens and differ from them mainly in stimulating protein synthesis at extragenital sites. Nandrolone decanoate (Deca-durabolin) is the only anabolic steroid studied in detail. Evidence suggests that anabolic steroids maintain or increase bone mass in women with osteoporosis, and weakly stimulate bone formation. However, androgenic and hepatic side effects and adverse lipoprotein changes virtually exclude their use in women.

In women who have had breast cancer, tamoxifen (an anti-oestrogen) seems nevertheless capable of preserving bone mass. The development of tamoxifen analogues, such as raloxifene, which apparently capable of increasing bone density without stimulating growth of the uterus or breast and which act as selective oestrogen receptor modulators, holds promise[30]. There is also some evidence that thiazide diuretics, which reduce urinary calcium excretion, may reduce fracture risk. New compounds under investigation include flavonoids such as ipriflavone.

Practical issues

Treatment of the patient with osteoporotic fracture

In theory, bone loss should be prevented before fractures occur; in real life, medical attention is sought only after the first fracture, often of the vertebra. One should not lose sight of the fact that the main (and only) reason for treating osteoporosis is to reduce fracture rate, and that the effectiveness of an antiresorptive agent should be judged by this.

In the patient with an apparently osteoporotic fracture, the important immediate steps are as follows:

- to establish the diagnosis
- to exclude any obvious secondary cause or risk factors
- to deal with immediate symptoms such as pain (with analgesics and back support)
- to explain the situation to the patient
- to formulate a plan of action (Figure 6.6).

Not all fractures are attributable to osteoporosis and especially in men other important causes such as myeloma need to be excluded (Chapter 4). If osteoporosis is present, there may be an obvious cause (secondary osteoporosis) or lifestyle risk factors (immobility, excessive smoking, excessive alcohol) (Chapter 4). A common clinical problem is a woman in the early menopause with her first vertebral fracture. The main aim is to prevent further bone loss. This means continuing mobility, avoiding deleterious lifestyle risk factors, taking sufficient oral calcium and making a decision about HRT or an alternative, such as a bisphosphonate.

For a woman who has had a hysterectomy, the cardiovascular and skeletal advantages of HRT probably outweigh the possible slight increase in breast cancer. For a woman with an intact uterus who needs progestogen, the advantages are less obvious and the side effects more troublesome.

HRT is most effective in maintaining bone mass in the early menopause, but it may be given both for treatment (i.e. after fracture) as

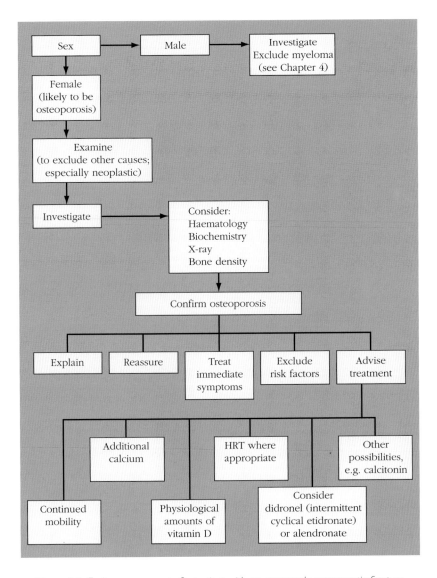

Figure 6.6 *Early management of a patient with an apparently osteoporotic fracture.*

well as for prevention (before fracture). The skeletal advantage of oestrogen is greatest during its administration and declines thereafter, and the rate of bone loss when oestrogen is stopped is probably similar to that just after the menopause. Thus, women aged 75–80 years who had a 10-year course of oestrogen that stopped 10–20 years earlier showed little difference in bone density from those who had not had oestrogen. Strategies can be devised to overcome this waning effect of oestrogen[31].

Where oestrogens are contraindicated (for example, where there is a personal history, or first-degree relative with a history of breast cancer, see Table 5.2) or where they are unacceptable, bisphosphonates should be considered, especially in elderly (more than 75 years) women. Cyclical etidronate is less expensive than alendronate, but may not be as effective at reducing limb fracture risk. However, alendronate has been associated with significant upper gastrointestinal toxicity.

Bone density measurement

The mean bone density in a population of hip fracture patients does not differ significantly from that of an age-matched non-fracture group and there is, therefore, little enthusiasm for population screening to detect those at risk of fracture. For each individual, however, a low bone density is the most important risk factor for future fracture (Chapter 4). Indications for bone densitometry (see Chapter 4, Table 4.3) include the following:

- oestrogen deficiency, corticosteroid use
- radiological osteopenia and vertebral deformity
- other fragility fractures
- monitoring treatment.

Thus, the accepted clinical indications for measurement of bone density include the assessment of bone mass as an indication of the likelihood of fracture, the exclusion (or otherwise) of osteopenia suspected on radiography and the investigation of patients with bone disease. Such measurements have introduced science to the skeleton, but their clinical application needs to be selective.

Falls

It has been emphasized that osteoporosis is only one factor influencing fracture, especially of the hip[1]. In the elderly, falls become increasingly more frequent as the benefits of previous HRT decline;

recent work emphasizes the importance of such falls and how their effect may be minimized[32]. Modulation of trauma to the skeleton may also be important. One trial has suggested that hip protectors worn by institutionalised elderly women could markedly reduce hip fracture incidence. Also in elderly patients, the propensity to hip fracture may depend more on simple geometry such as hip axis length (the distance from greater trochanter to inner pelvic brim) than on BMD[33]. Despite this the maintenance of bone mass remains a priority for prevention, and ideally should start early in life and not when age and falls have already wreaked skeletal havoc.

Other causes of osteoporosis

Most osteoporotic fractures occur in postmenopausal women; thus, osteoporosis at this age has received most investigation. Osteoporosis in men, or that due to corticosteroid therapy, however, should not be neglected; rare forms of osteoporosis, such as osteogenesis imperfecta and idiopathic juvenile osteoporosis, may also cause problems (Chapter 4).

In summary, the treatment as well as the prevention of osteoporosis depends on the intelligent application of the known facts about bone cell biology. Provided that secondary causes and risk factors have been dealt with, the maintenance of the skeleton depends on its continued mechanical use, sufficient calcium intake and appropriate hormone replacement (Figure 6.7). There is also some evidence that adding calcium or etidronate to an HRT regimen increases the beneficial skeletal effect of HRT alone, at least to certain parts of the skeleton[34,35].

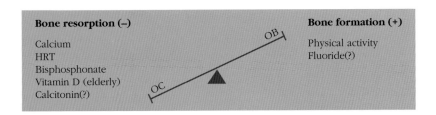

Figure 6.7 *Scheme for the preservation of the skeleton. OC = osteoclasts; OB = osteoblasts.*

115

Key points

▓ The treatment of osteoporosis deals with the skeleton when significant bone loss has already occurred.

▓ Treatment attempts to reverse the imbalance between bone formation and bone resorption.

▓ Since it is difficult to increase bone formation, treatment of osteoporosis largely depends on reducing bone resorption.

▓ The effect of antiresorptive therapy is limited by the state of the bone, its rate of turnover and the agent used.

▓ In practice, the prevention of further bone loss depends on the avoidance of known risk factors and a combination of exercise, additional calcium and (where appropriate) hormone replacement therapy (HRT). Where HRT is inappropriate or unacceptable, bisphosphonates provide a useful non-hormonal alternative.

References

1 Riggs L, Melton LJ. The prevention and treatment of osteoporosis. *N Eng J Med* 1992; **327**: 620–7.

2 Dempster DW, Lindsay R. Pathogenesis of osteoporosis. *Lancet* 1993; **341**: 797–801.

3 Lindsay R. Prevention and treatment of osteoporosis. *Lancet* 1993; **341**: 801–5.

4 Smith R. Prevention and treatment of osteoporosis: common sense and science coincide. *J Bone Joint Surg* 1994; **76B** 345–7.

5 Marcus R, Feldman D, Kelsey J, eds. *Osteoporosis*. New York: Academic Press, 1996.

6 Compston JE. Structural mechanisms of trabecular bone loss. In: Smith R, ed. *Osteoporosis 1990*. London: RCP Publications, 1990; 35–43.

7 Snow CM, Matrin CC, Shaw JM. Physical activity and the risk for osteoporosis. In: Marcus R, Feldman D, Kelsey J, eds. *Osteoporosis*. New York: Academic Press, 1996; 511–28.

8 Riggs BL, Hodgson SF, O'Fallon WM *et al*. Effect of fluoride treatment on the fracture rate in postmenopausal women with osteoporosis. *N Engl J Med* 1990; **322**: 802–9.

9 Pak CYC, Sakhaee K, Adams-Huet B *et al*. Treatment of post-menopausal osteoporosis with slow-release sodium fluoride. *Ann Intern Med* 1995; **123**: 401–8.

10 Mundy GR. No bones about fluoride. *Nature Med* 1995; **1**: 1130–1.

11 Finkelstein JS, Klibanski A, Schaeffer EH *et al*. Parathyroid hormone for the prevention of bone loss induced by estrogen deficiency. *N Engl J Med* 1994; **331**: 1618–23.

12 Grady D, Rubin SM, Petitti DB *et al*. Hormone therapy to prevent disease and prolong life in postmenopausal women. *Ann Intern Med* 1992; **117**: 1106–37.

13 Birge SJ, Mortel KF. Estrogen and the treatment of Alzheimer's disease. *Am J Med* 1997; **103**: 365–455.

14 Davidson NE. Hormone replacement therapy — breast versus heart versus bone. *N Engl J Med* 1995; **332**: 1638–9.

15 Vandenbroucke JP, Helmerhorst FM. Risk of venous thrombosis with hormone replacement therapy. *Lancet* 1996; **348**: 972.

16 Heaney RP. Thinking straight about calcium. *N Engl J Med* 1993; **328**: 503–5.

17 Dawson-Hughes B. The role of calcium in the treatment of osteoporosis. In: Marcus R, Feldman D, Kelsey J, eds. *Osteoporosis*. New York: Academic Press, 1996; 1159–68.

18 Chapuy MC, Arlott ME, Duboeuf F *et al*. Vitamin D₃ and calcium to prevent hip fractures in elderly women. *N Engl J Med* 1992; **327**: 1637–42.

19 Johnston CC, Miller JZ, Reister TK *et al*. Calcium supplements and increases in bone mineral density in children. *N Engl J Med* 1992; **327**: 82–7.

20 Lloyd T, Andon MB, Rollings RN *et al*. Calcium supplementation and bone mineral density in adolescent girls. *JAMA* 1993; **270**: 841–4.

21 Prince RL, Smith M, Dick IM *et al*. Prevention of postmenopausal osteoporosis. A comparative study of exercise, calcium supplementation and hormone replacement therapy. *N Engl J Med* 1991; **325**: 1189–95.

22 Matkovic V. Calcium intake and peak bone mass. *N Engl J Med* 1992; **327**: 119–20.

23 Marcus R. Cyclic etidronate: has the rose lost its bloom? *Am J Med* 1993; **95**: 555–6.

24 Storm T, Kollerup G, Thamsborg G *et al*. Five years of clinical experience with intermittent cyclical etidronate for post-menopausal osteoporosis. *J Rheumatol* 1996; **23**: 1560–4.

25 Liberman UA, Weiss SR, Broll J *et al*. Effect of oral alendronate on bone mineral density and the incidence of fractures in postmenopausal osteoporosis. The Alendronate Phase III Osteoporosis Treatment Study Group. *N Eng J Med* 1995; **333**: 1437–43.

26 Black DM, Cummings SR, Karpf DB *et al*. Randomised trial of effect of alendronate on risk of fracture in women with existing vertebral fractures. *Lancet* 1996; **348**: 1535–41.

27 Dawson-Hughes B, Dallal GE, Krall EA *et al*. Effect of vitamin D supplementation on wintertime and overall bone loss in healthy postmenopausal women. *Ann Intern Med* 1991; **115**: 505–12.

28 Reid IR. Vitamin D and its metabolites in the management of osteoporosis. In: Marcus R, Feldman D, Kelsey J, eds. *Osteoporosis*. New York: Academic Press, 1996; 1169–90.

29 Christiansen C. Androgens and androgenic progestins. In: Marcus R, Feldman D, Kelsey J, eds. *Osteoporosis*. New York: Academic Press, 1996; 1279–92.

30 Short L, Glasebrook AL, Adrian MD *et al*. Distinct effect of selective oestrogen receptor modulators on oestrogen dependent and oestrogen independent human breast cancer cell proliferation. *J Bone Min Res* 1996; 11 (Suppl.): S482 (abstr).

31 Ettinger B, Grady D. The waning effect of postmenopausal estrogen therapy in osteoporosis. *N Engl J Med* 1993; **329**: 1192–3.

32 Province MA, Hadley EC, Hornbrook MC *et al.* The effects of exercise on falls in elderly patients. A preplanned meta-analysis of the FICSIT trials. Frailty and Injuries: Cooperative Studies of Intervention Techniques. *JAMA* 1995; **273**: 1341–7.

33 Faulkner KG, McClung M, Cummings SR. Automated evaluation of hip axis length for predicting hip fracture. *J Bone Min Res* 1994; **9**: 1065–70.

34 Haines CJ, Chung TKH, Leung PC *et al.* Calcium supplementation and bone mineral density in postmenopausal women using estrogen replacement therapy. *Bone* 1995; **16**: 529–31.

35 Wimalawansa SJ. Combined therapy with estrogen and etidronate has an additive effect on bone mineral density in the hip and vertebrae: four year randomised study. *Am J Med* 1995; **99**: 36–42.

Chapter 7

Current problems

Introduction

Advances in the prevention and treatment of osteoporosis and, most importantly, in the prevention of fracture, will depend, in the final analysis, on a better understanding of cell biology. In theory, it should be possible to develop bone-sparing agents aimed precisely at the bone cells, ideally to increase bone formation, but the practical difficulties are considerable.

One increasingly used measure of the effectiveness of such agents will be a reduced rate of loss or a gain in measured bone mineral density (BMD), but the relationship of this to bone architecture, strength and fracture rate is complex and requires further investigation.

Not all forms of osteoporosis are the same since, even within the postmenopausal group, there is a spectrum of disease and, for this reason, treatments need to be individual and not wholesale.

Amongst the clinical problems outlined in the recent AGO report[1] is the development of health care strategies to ensure that patients receive the most effective assistance for their skeletal problems. This is the aim of shared health care (Chapter 8).

Current problems are dealt with under question headings. The reader will realize that the effective management of osteoporosis is not simple.

What are the problems of bone cell biology?

These are innumerable[2]. We have some idea of where bone cells come from and what they do (Chapter 2), but we have very little idea of how they 'talk' to each other. Legions of putative cellular messengers (cytokines) are described, but nearly all research is conducted *in vitro* on cells of dubious derivation and little applies *in vivo* to the human skeleton. Despite this — and since we must start somewhere — it remains important to unravel the nature of the linkage between the osteoblast and osteoclast, as these so-called 'coupling factors' are likely to be central to skeletal biology.

During the formation of the organic matrix of bone, osteoblasts synthesize growth-regulatory factors such as insulin-like growth factor (IGF-1), the bone morphogenetic proteins (BMPs) and other members of the transforming growth factor beta (TGF-β) family (Chapter 2). It is suggested that, during osteoclast-mediated resorption of bone, these growth factors are released locally to stimulate osteoblast activity; this is one aspect of coupling[3]. Another aspect involves the production by the osteoblasts of so-called osteoclast-differentiation factors that recognize osteoclast precursors and prepare them to differentiate into mature osteoclasts[4]. It has also been demonstrated that bone marrow-derived stromal cells produce soluble factors, such as macrophage colony-stimulating factor (M-CSF), that act on osteoclasts throughout their development.

Clearly, the development of new osteotropic agents (below) should take into account this 'coupling' of cellular activity, since the main property of such an agent must be to bring about uncoupling in favour of formation. It has been proposed that growth factors and BMPs could be used to do this[5]. In the current enthusiasm for osteoclasts and osteoblasts one must not forget the humble osteocyte. If, as some believe, this living cell in mineralized bone transforms mechanical signals into cytokines that mediate the appropriate cellular responses (in this instance the formation of new bone where mechanical stimuli are greatest), the identification of these biochemical messages could be of equal importance to the putative coupling factors.

What is the relation between bone mass, density and strength?

The aim of managing osteoporosis is to restore bone strength and to reduce fracture rate. For expediency, the efficiency of an anti-osteoporotic regime is most often assessed by measuring the BMD rather than the fracture rate. This gives a false sense of security: BMD is not a true density (being expressed as gCa/cm^2) and measures bone mineral only; it gives no idea about the structure and composition of the bone within which this mineral lives. Despite this, there is a comforting inverse statistical relationship between BMD and fracture rate. This is not strictly linear and a therapeutically induced increase in bone density can be associated with disproportionate decrease in fracture rate.

It is clear that the current DXA measurements of BMD, useful though they are, have limitations. For this reason, methods such as ultrasound are of increasing interest, not least because they provide indirect information about structure as well as amount.

What is the appropriate clinical use of bone density or related measurements?

The current clinical indications for DXA densitometry have been discussed (Chapter 4). Controversy arises mainly because of its expense (in comparison to other routine biochemical and radiological measurements), and its relevance to the only important clinical outcome, i.e. fracture.

It has been pointed out (page 32) that there is a close parallel to the relationship between plasma cholesterol measurement and ischaemic heart disease (IHD). It is relatively easy to demonstrate the direct relationship between circulating cholesterol concentration and IHD and inversely between BMD and fracture rate. What is less easy to demonstrate is that reducing cholesterol reduces IHD, and that increasing BMD reduces fracture rate: in both the cholesterol and BMD models there is a considerable overlap between populations, so that those who have IHD do not all have abnormally high cholesterol levels and in those who have fractures the BMD overlaps with those who do not. This second point is one important reason why epidemiologists oppose population screening, i.e. the measurement of BMD throughout populations, in order to identify those with a low BMD who are more likely to suffer a fracture than those with a normal BMD. Nevertheless, measurement of BMD by DXA is the only method that quantifies the amount of bone within the skeleton (conventionally expressed as 'bone density') and, for this reason, it might be more widely used if it were not so expensive (in comparison, for instance, to the measurement of cholesterol). It is worth challenging this assumption. The current indications for bone density measurement — as a baseline before starting perimenopausal or postmenopausal hormone replacement therapy (HRT), as a way of excluding radiological osteopenia, as an indication of the effectiveness (or otherwise) of treatment, and in the assessment of subjects at risk of osteoporosis — are unlikely to increase unless population screening becomes epidemiologically and economically acceptable. The measurement of BMD in patients with primary hyperparathyroidism is a rare but accepted indication for densitometry, as a low bone density may be considered an indication for parathyroidectomy.

The proper role of densitometry is not yet firmly established. The general practitioner and the consultant should decide between them when knowledge of bone density is likely to influence management, and when it is not.

How important are so-called risk factors in determining skeletal outcome?

As the main measurable determinant of fracture risk is BMD, those factors that contribute to a low bone density are, in general, those that contribute to fracture[6]. This statement necessarily excludes falls, accidents and trauma, which can cause fracture without pre-existing low bone density.

Race (BMD is lower in White Caucasians and Orientals than in Blacks) and family history (in first-degree relatives) are important genetic determinants of bone density. BMD is also related to the number of reproductive years and is reduced by oestrogen deficiency, excessive thinness and (in females) excessive exercise. Of lifestyle factors, smoking probably significantly reduces BMD, whereas alcohol (unless very excessive) has little effect. The distinction between risk factors for low bone density and the causes of secondary osteoporosis is poorly defined. Likewise, the results of large series that attempt to identify risk factors for osteoporosis do not always agree. In practice, it is usual to enquire about all the factors likely to contribute to osteoporosis, but experience shows that, for individuals, the measured BMD does not always agree with that suggested by a risk-factor history.

What is the role of biochemistry in treatment decisions?

Outside the research environment, biochemical measurements are useful only to exclude other bone diseases masquerading as osteoporosis and to identify the causes of secondary osteoporosis. Treatment decisions are rarely influenced by such simple indications of excess bone resorption as increased urine calcium, and it has not been shown convincingly that biochemical measurements either relate to BMD or predict the rate of bone loss in individuals. However, in some women with postmenopausal osteoporosis, bone turnover (measured biochemically) is increased; it might be expected, therefore, that these women would lose bone more rapidly than those with a less rapid bone turnover, and would therefore be more susceptible to fractures in subsequent years.

The proposal is that if it were possible to identify these 'high-turnover fast losers' (and if they were, indeed, those with a subsequent low bone density and increased fracture rate), then this would help with treatment decisions. Further, if this identification could be by simple biochemical means (which could be repeated when necessary), then it would be worthwhile.

Much work has now gone into this problem. It has been mainly concerned with the crosslinked collagen-derived peptides (Chapter 4), where changes in bone resorption in osteoporosis may be detected more easily than by other methods. At present there is no convincing evidence that, for an individual (and possibly even for groups), measurement of these peptides will alter clinical decision making.

Do all forms of osteoporosis need the same treatment?

This book concentrates on osteoporosis in postmenopausal women because of its frequency and complications. However, the secondary forms of osteoporosis are also important because in some of them the underlying cause is treatable (Chapter 4), for instance in thyrotoxicosis, coeliac disease and hypogonadism. It is clear that the treatment of osteoporosis should be individual, both within the postmenopausal group and outside it. One of the most important forms of osteoporosis is that induced by corticosteroids. The bone biology of this form differs from that of the menopause, since the primary effect of corticosteroids is to suppress osteoblastic activity. This, combined with a temporary increase in bone resorption, leads to uncoupling of these bone cell activities (analogous to acute immobilization in the young) with a rapid loss of bone that is difficult to treat and requires specialist attention. Osteoporosis also occurs in men, often without a readily identifiable cause. Deficiency of testosterone is detectable in a significant proportion of men with osteoporosis and corticosteroid use is also an important risk factor.

What is the long-term effect of antiresorptive drugs, and what happens when they are stopped?

For the purposes of these questions, the main agents are HRT and the bisphosphonates. They act on bone in different ways and our knowledge about them is incomplete.

The advantages and disadvantages of HRT have been discussed (Chapters 5 and 6): the former include preservation of the skeleton, and reduction of cardiovascular mortality; the latter include increase in cancer of the breast and endometrium, and probably of thromboembolism. It is likely that these effects diminish when HRT is discontinued. One important point is how rapidly this subsequent bone loss occurs, but there is little information on this. When HRT is first given to a postmenopausal woman, the BMD increases quite rapidly in the first year (by about 5–10%) and less so in the second. In general, the BMD is maintained or falls slightly as long as HRT is given, but falls quite rapidly as soon as therapy is stopped. Current evidence suggests that the initial rate of fall may be equal to the initial rate of gain when HRT is first given, or approximately the same rate as in the early postmenopausal years. Whatever the cause of this, the outcome would be that, several years after stopping HRT, the skeletal benefits (as judged by BMD) would be lost. If this were confirmed, it would constitute a major problem in the use of HRT.

For bisphosphonates the problems are different. These compounds do not have the non-skeletal advantages and disadvantages of HRT. Apart from high-dose etidronate, they do not carry the risk of interference with mineralization. One theoretical long-term effect of the powerful new bisphosphonates is the possibility of causing a sustained suppression of the bone cells. Such an effect would be likely to interfere with the bone multicellular units and the self-repair mechanism of normal bone, leading to increased fragility. Further, since bisphosphonates are selectively incorporated into bone tissue for a long time, such an effect on bone strength could persist for years after the bisphosphonate was discontinued. Animal studies suggest that this does not occur, and there is no evidence of it in humans, but the length of treatment with powerful new bisphosphonates has been relatively short. There is some evidence that bone loss may be rapid when bisphosphonates (in this example pamidronate) are stopped[7].

What sort of osteotropic agents should we be developing?

In the management of osteoporosis there are 'common sense' measures that should be continued as a background to more potentially dramatic advances, unless they are found to be positively dangerous. Such measures include exercise, plenty of calcium, physiological amounts of vitamin D and the avoidance of risk factors. But where will osteotropic advances come from?

There are two clear possibilities: the first is the development of currently used drugs, such as oestrogens and bisphosphonates, that reduce bone resorption; the second is the development of new drugs, such as growth factors and morphogenetic proteins, potentially capable of stimulating bone formation.

Amongst bisphosphonates, modification of the side chains to increase potency and antiresorbing specificity is likely to continue, with the major difficulty being very low and variable oral absorption. Amongst oestrogens much needs to be done to increase their acceptability. The development of oestrogen-related compounds that have tissue-selective effects on the oestrogen receptor should be of considerable importance, removing the disadvantages of oestrogen (due to its effect on the uterus and possibly on breast tissue) while retaining the skeletal, cardiovascular (and possibly nervous system) advantages.

However, only a limited skeletal benefit comes from blocking bone resorption (for reasons explained in Chapters 2 and 6) and an ideal drug for management of osteoporosis would be one that has a specific effect on the osteoblast. Such a drug would need to be acceptable (preferably by mouth) to the patient, should have no significant side effects and should produce a controlled increase in the amount of normal bone. No current drug fits these criteria.

Candidates include growth factors, such as IGF-1, parathyroid hormone fragments, BMPs and members of the TGF-β family. All these agents have widespread effects outside the skeleton: as an example, the BMPs are so named because they can cause extraskeletal ossification.

Even if it were possible to produce an increase in the amount of bone by stimulating osteoblast activity, this is not the whole answer — as indicated by the effect of sodium fluoride, where the new bone tissue is not normal. There is also the theoretical possibility that an increase in osteoblastic activity would be paralleled by an increase in osteoclastic activity, producing a high turnover, dense, but fragile bone (by analogy with Paget's disease).

The future

Although the apparent aims of bone cell biologists, physicians and orthopaedic surgeons differ widely, they are all concerned with understanding the control of the amount and strength of bone. For the future, the most important achievement would be the prevention of structural failure and the reduction of fracture rate. This will not be done easily. It will mean increasing the strength of bone and decreasing the rate of injury predominantly from falls in later years. Significant advances will require much financial support.

Key points

■ The development of new methods to control bone mass depends on advances in knowledge of bone biology.

■ The efficacy of such methods should ideally be based on the reduction of fracture rate rather than on changes in BMD.

■ Advances in cell biology and clinical research in bone should be used to afford the patient maximum benefit.

■ In order for this to occur, an efficient system of shared care of osteoporotic patients is necessary (Chapter 8).

References

1 *Report of the Advisory Group on Osteoporosis.* Report on Osteoporosis. Wetherby: Department of Health, 1994.

2 Bilezikan JP, Raisz LG, Rodan GA. *Principles of Bone Biology.* San Diego: Academic Press, 1996.

3 Hayden JM, Mohan S, Baylink DJ. The insulin-like growth factor system and the coupling of formation to resorption. *Bone* 1995; **17**: 93S–98S (Suppl. 2).

4 Suda T, Udagawa N, Nakamura I, Miyaura C, Takahashi N. Modulation of osteoclast differentiation by local factors. *Bone* 1995; **17**: 87S–91S (Suppl. 2).

5 Seeman E, Tsalamandris C, Bass S, Pearce G. Present and future of osteoporosis therapy. *Bone* 1995; **17**: 23S–29S (Suppl.)

6 Cummings SR, Nevitt MC, Browner WS *et al.* Risk factors for hip fracture in white women. Study of Osteoporotic Fractures Research Group. *N Engl J Med* 1995; **332**: 767–73.

7 Orr-Walker B, Wattie DJ, Evans MC, Reid IR. Effects of prolonged bisphosphonate therapy and its discontinuation on bone mineral density in post-menopausal osteoporosis. *Clin Endocrinol* 1997; **46**: 87–92.

Chapter 8

Implications for shared care

Introduction

'Shared care for osteoporosis' describes the joint management of osteoporosis by general practitioners supported by a primary health care team, and hospital doctors supported by a hospital-based infrastructure. When considering this shared approach to patient management, it becomes clear that a large variety of medical and paramedical staff may be involved at different stages of the disease process, and that management will vary accordingly. However, the overall purpose remains to provide the most appropriate patient care to the greatest number, given the resources that are available. A unified approach should avoid unnecessary investigation and treatment while preserving resources for those in greatest need. It should maximize the ability of primary care to meet the needs of the majority (Tables 8.1 and 8.2).

The health care challenge

While the health problems caused by osteoporosis are currently sizeable (Chapter 3), projection to the middle of the twenty-first century is alarming. In the USA today there are about four people in work for every retired person. In 50 years' time, the population over the age of 65 years will have almost tripled and the population over 85 years will have increased six-fold. Considering that 95% of hip fractures in women occur in those over the age of 65 (Hospital

Table 8.1 Hospital clinicians who regularly have contact with osteoporotic patients or those at increased risk of bone loss

■ Orthopaedic surgeons

■ Gynaecologists

■ General (and other) physicians

■ Rheumatologists

■ Endocrinologists

■ Metabolic medicine specialists

■ Biochemists

■ Radiologists

Inpatient Enquiry data 1985), osteoporosis-related fractures, if left unchecked, are likely to become a huge and unaffordable drain on scarce health care resources[1].

Most of those who will be at greatest risk in 50 years time are alive now and possess their peak bone mass. There is, therefore, considerable opportunity over the next few years to modify bone loss in this cohort. Consideration of how this might be done in a cost-effective way should be given high priority.

Given the magnitude of the current and potential problem, general practitioners will necessarily be the principal group of doctors to provide most patient care. If these generalists are to provide high standards of care to patients, they must ensure that they themselves are adequately trained and that they have the necessary human and material resources to identify patients at risk, to investigate them appropriately, and to advise, treat and refer those cases to the appropriate consultant service available to them.

Table 8.2 Contributors to osteoporosis care in the community

Description	Role
District Nurses	Care of patients at home after fracture Advice to women after hysterectomy Dietary advice to the elderly Identification of those at high risk Avoidance of falls in the elderly
Practice Nurses	Health promotion, diet, exercise Identification of those at high risk Advice on treatment options
Dietitians	Dietary advice (all ages); vitamin and mineral supplementation
Health visitors	Health promotion; diet and exercise; special responsibility for the young
Pharmacists	Vitamin and mineral supplementation; drug treatment advice
Physiotherapists	Fracture rehabilitation; pain reduction; maintenance of mobility
Occupational therapists	Maintenance of mobility and independence
Medical practitioners	Health promotion Identification of those at high risk of osteoporosis Prevention of bone loss in 'at risk' individuals Investigation and diagnosis Referral of relevant cases to consultant care Short- and long-term management

Figure 8.1 depicts the interfaces and describes the functions of those involved in an osteoporosis service. This service will coexist with those already in place for the provision of fracture management, rehabilitation, parallel conditions and others.

Mechanisms of shared care

A hospital service should be led by a clinician with a special interest in osteoporosis. In different regions the background of this person will vary but osteoporosis is unlikely to be the sole interest of such a clinician. Osteoporosis should not be considered to be the sole domain of a single medical discipline. The lead clinician should collaborate with primary care physicians and agree with them on local guidelines for the provision of osteoporosis services.

The lead clinician should oversee the provision of bone density measurement, but this and other necessary investigations (Chapter 4) should be directly available to general practitioners, wherever possible.

Currently (1996), access to bone densitometry is patchy. There are only 90 dual X-ray absorptiometry (DXA) machines in the UK and only

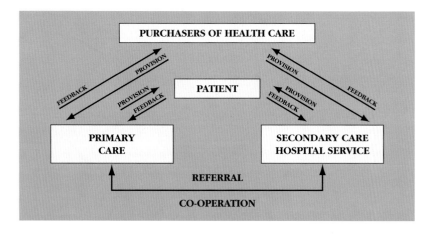

Figure 8.1 *Relationship between patients, purchasers and providers, for the optimal management of osteoporosis.*

12% have been purchased by health authorities[2]. The UK lags behind nearly every other developed country in this respect (Figure 8.2).

The principal determinants of health care provision within a geographical area are the available human and material resources. The nature of shared care in osteoporosis varies accordingly; in some areas no specific service exists, whereas in others it is well developed. Dissemination of 'best care' to those that have no provision for osteoporosis must be the first priority.

Osteoporosis is a rapidly developing subject that necessitates frequent information transfer between physicians. In many areas where a hospital-based service exists, it is often relatively new and will need to evolve and be responsive to the rapidly changing needs and expectations of the population that it serves. Continuous assessment of new technology and treatments is needed for efficient resource allocation. Shared care should foster closer understanding and agreement about the provision of care in a locality, as well as early dissemination of new research findings.

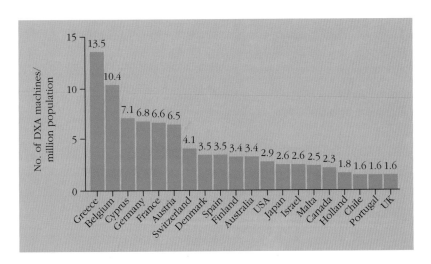

Figure 8.2 *Histogram of the number of DXA machines per million population in different countries. (Reproduced from ref. 2, with permission.)*

Although the title of this book relates principally to the shared responsibilities of doctors in primary and secondary care, it is clear that the complex nature of the problems that are attributable to osteoporosis, and that an individual may face, requires a multidisciplinary approach.

Key points

■ Current provision of services for those with osteoporosis or at risk of developing osteoporosis is suboptimal.

■ Demands upon services will increase and funding needs to reflect this.

■ A locally developed and applied model of shared responsibility for the care of those with osteoporosis is likely to be the most effective method of health care delivery.

References

1 Royal College of Physicians report 'Fractured neck of femur, prevention and management' 1989.

2 Advisory Group on Osteoporosis. *Report on Osteoporosis.* Wetherby: Department of Health, 1994.

Index